exercise your way to health:
arthritis

exercise plans to improve your life

Paula Coates

National Rheumatoid
Arthritis Society

B L O O M S B U R Y
LONDON · OXFORD · NEW YORK · NEW DELHI · SYDNEY

Published in 2010 by
Bloomsbury Sport
An imprint of Bloomsbury Publishing Plc
50 Bedford Square, London WC1B 3DP, UK
www.bloomsbury.com

Reprinted 2017

ISBN 978 14081 0702 7

A CIP catalogue record for this book is available from the British Library.

Acknowledgements
Cover photograph © Shutterstock
Inside photographs © Grant Pritchard, except pp 4, 10, 20, 41, 43, 56, 77 Shutterstock, p80 iStockphotos.com
Illustrations by Jeff Edwards
Designed by James Watson
Commissioned by Charlotte Croft
Edited by Kate Turvey

This book is produced using paper that is made from wood grown in managed, sustainable forests. It is natural, renewable and recyclable. The logging and manufacturing processes conform to the environmental regulations of the country of origin.

Typeset in 9.25pt AGaramond on 12pt by Margaret Brain.

Printed and bound in India by Replika Press Pvt. Ltd.

contents

acknowledgements

I would like to say a big thank you to all those who have given their time and support to me during the writing of this book – family, friends, and colleagues alike. A special thank you to all my patients who have been my greatest teachers and have allowed their experiences to be included in this book. Finally, a big thank you to Charlotte Croft and Kate Turvey at A&C Black, my models and Grant Pritchard for his photography.

foreword

I have lived with severe rheumatoid arthritis (RA) for nearly 30 years. To say that this has been challenging and at times overwhelming is understating the impact that this painful, chronic and incurable disease can have on your life and the lives of your family, friends and colleagues.

However, I found that when I started to learn more about my disease and its complications and tried putting into practice various self-management and coping strategies, I felt more in control and more at ease with my problems, and more able to face whatever the future threw at me.

We now know from research that those who are positive in outlook and apply the principles of self-management, generally enjoy a better quality of life and achieve better long-term outcomes. With this in mind, learning more about your disease is a real investment in your health. Self-management helps you to manage your pain and flare-ups by strategies such as pacing, relaxation and goal-setting. Building suitable exercise into your normal routine is also extremely important and this book will give you lots of good information.

Today's therapies and approach to RA treatment are so much more effective than they were when I was diagnosed. I am sure you will find this book helpful. Good luck.

Ailsa Bosworth
Founder and Chief Executive
National Rheumatoid Arthritis Society

endorsement

As a busy working GP and musculoskeletal specialist I can highly recommend this book as essential reading for patients and clinicians alike. This book is well researched, concise and up-to-date, and written by a first rate, highly experienced physiotherapist. It will give much needed and added support for patients diagnosed with either osteo-arthritis or rheumatoid arthritis who want to do all they can to understand and manage their condition.

Dr Gregor McEwan MB BS Dip Sports Med Lon

introduction

The management of chronic conditions such as rheumatoid arthritis and osteoarthritis has been a part of my everyday working life as a physiotherapist for the past 14 years. I have specialised in caring for people with arthritis after working in some of the leading rheumatological units in the country, helping people manage their symptoms, return to work and improve their physical fitness. In this book I will tell you what I have learnt from my patients over the years and what I know will help you manage your joint pain, stay active and improve your health and fitness.

Osteoarthritis is extremely common, and can develop as part of the ageing process for all of us. About 1 per cent of the world's population is affected by rheumatoid arthritis and women are three times more likely to develop it than men. Whatever your diagnosis, you may be feeling anxious about what the future holds. All this is understandable and this book aims to help you pick up what you need to know about both these conditions, to allow you to make the choices that are best for you.

This book will:
- teach you the facts about osteoarthritis and rheumatoid arthritis
- dispel the myths about arthritis
- show you how to manage your arthritis in the flare-up and non flare-up phases
- give you an exercise programme to build into your lifestyle
- help you understand and avoid the stress and anxiety associated with chronic pain
- allow you to get on with your everyday life.

The book is split into three main parts. **Part 1** covers the basics that you need to know about your condition. It includes answers to all the questions you might wish you had asked the doctor, but didn't ask because you were busy taking on board the fact that you had just received your diagnosis. Once you know exactly what you are dealing with, it is much easier to manage and formulate a plan to move yourself forward with your life.

Part 2 looks at what you can do to help yourself: the changes you can make to your lifestyle that will help you become fitter, healthier and in control of your own health. It is all too easy to feel out of control when you have just been diagnosed, and this book aims to help you get that control back. There is also information on the best places to go for such advice.

Part 3 covers the exercises that you can use to strengthen your body, maintain full range of movement in your joints and help prevent further problems. Prevention is always better than cure, and usually much less painful. I will show you the exercises that will help you return to fitness no matter how unfit you are now. I will also show you how to monitor your own progress with simple tests that you can perform at home. When you see the results of adding exercise to your life you will wish you had done it sooner.

As you read through the book you will see I have used a traffic light system of treatment options. This is designed to make it easy for you to see the options available to you at a glance and to tell when you will need to see a specialist.

The traffic lights work as follows:

Green	Amber	Red
Go ahead: you can start self treatment immediately to manage your disease and prevent it from becoming worse.	**Proceed with caution:** you may need assessment and treatments that a physiotherapist or health care professional may advise to manage your flare-up.	**Stop!** Things are serious and need assessment to rule out complications and you may need to take advice on the best way to manage things this time.

what can I do if I have arthritis?

Millions of people live with long-term conditions such as rheumatoid and osteoarthritis. Most of them lead a full and active life by adapting their lifestyles in response to their symptoms. By increasing your understanding of the condition and how you can help yourself to health, you can improve the quality of your life.

Arthritis can affect your health over a long period of time, possibly your entire life, and in many cases there is no cure. When you are first diagnosed it is easy to feel overwhelmed and as if the condition has taken over your life, especially if you need to take medication on a daily basis. It's important to understand that your condition can become a serious problem. However, you can take steps to control the negative effects of arthritis and inflammatory joint disease on your health.

One method of taking control is 'self-management'. Self-management allows you take responsibility for doing what it takes to manage your illness effectively. Your doctor, nurse and physiotherapist can make treatment recommendations, but they won't make a difference unless you choose to follow their advice. There is always more than one treatment plan, as what works best for one person won't necessarily work best for you. Talking about the different treatment options available will help you create and choose a plan that is right for you. If you take control in this way, you will start to feel motivated to make changes to your lifestyle and engage in active self-management. When you take care of your body, it will take care of you and help prevent problems in the future.

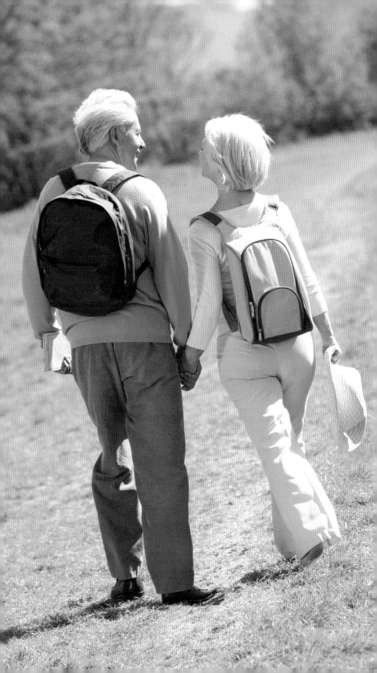

part 1

understanding arthritis

osteoarthritis

what is osteoarthritis?

Osteoarthritis is sometimes called 'wear and tear' or 'degenerative joint disease'. It is the most common form of arthritis and occurs when the cartilage in your joints becomes thinned over time, or extra bone is laid down around the joint in response to injury or strain. Osteoarthritis can affect any joint in your body, although it most commonly affects joints in your hands, hips, knees and spine. Typically it affects just one joint, but, as with arthritis of the fingers, several joints can be affected.

Osteoarthritis gradually worsens over time, and no cure exists. It is a natural side-effect of ageing, just like grey hair and wrinkles, and in the same way some people will be affected more than others. There are treatments that can relieve pain and help you remain active. By taking steps to exercise you can actively manage your osteoarthritis and gain control over the associated pain.

signs and symptoms

The progression of the bony changes associated with osteoarthritis is slow. The symptoms also develop slowly and worsen over time. The list below outlines the most common symptoms and when you are most likely to notice them.

- **pain** in a joint during or after use, or after a period of inactivity.

- **swelling** – in some cases but not always.

- **tenderness** in the joint when you apply light pressure.

- **stiffness** in and around a joint, which may be most noticeable when you first wake up in the morning or after a period of inactivity.

- **loss of flexibility**, which may make it difficult to use the joint for normal functional tasks.

- **grating sensation** when you move the joint.

- **bone spurs**, which appear as hard lumps, can form around the affected joint and are seen clearly on X-rays.

Although most commonly felt in the hands, hips, knees and spine, it is possible to develop arthritis in other joints, especially if you have been injured or placed unusual stress on a joint. It is uncommon for osteoarthritis to affect your jaw, shoulder, elbows, wrists or ankles, but it is possible if you have sustained a fracture or played a sport that has increased the stress through a particular joint.

what causes osteoarthritis?

Osteoarthritis occurs when the cartilage covering the ends of bones in your joints becomes thinner over time. The smooth surface of the cartilage becomes rough, causing irritation. Eventually, if the cartilage wears down completely, the surface ends of your bones become worn and your joints become painful. This additional pressure on the bones can make them swell.

In most cases it isn't clear what causes osteoarthritis, but research has shown that it's a combination of things, including being overweight, ageing, joint injury or stress, family history and muscle weakness.

The most likely causes are:

- **Age:** osteoarthritis typically occurs in older adults. People under 40 rarely experience osteoarthritis.

- **Sex:** women are more likely to develop osteoarthritis, though it isn't clear why.

- **Bone deformities:** some people are born with joint deformities or defective cartilage, which may increase the risk of osteoarthritis.

- **Joint injuries:** injuries that occur when playing sports, or from an accident, may increase the risk of developing osteoarthritis.

- **Obesity:** carrying more body weight places more stress on your weight-bearing joints, such as your knees.

- **Other diseases that affect the bones and joints:** diseases that increase the risk of osteoarthritis include gout, rheumatoid arthritis, Paget's disease of bone and septic arthritis.

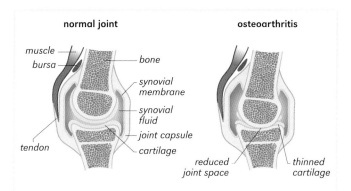

Figure 1.1 A normal knee joint compared to a knee joint with osteoarthritis – the thinning of the cartilage and the inflamed synovial membrane and how this creates swelling in the joint

when to seek medical advice

⬤ If you have swelling or stiffness in your joints that lasts for more than two weeks, make an appointment with your doctor. If you're already taking medication for osteoarthritis, contact your doctor if you're experiencing side-effects from your arthritis medications. Tell your doctor if you experience side-effects such as nausea, abdominal discomfort, black or tarry stools, constipation, or drowsiness.

screening and diagnosis

If your doctor suspects you have osteoarthritis, he or she will examine your affected joint and ask you questions about your joint pain. To find out more about what is causing your pain, your doctor may also recommend some tests:

- **X-rays:** X-rays of your joints may reveal a narrowing of the space within a joint, which indicates that the cartilage is thinning. An X-ray may also show bone spurs around a joint (see page 9).

- **Blood tests:** Blood tests may help rule out other causes of joint pain, such as rheumatoid arthritis or infection.

- **Joint fluid analysis:** Your doctor may use a long needle to draw fluid out of the affected joint. Testing the fluid can determine whether your pain is caused by gout (see box opposite) or an infection, or whether it is osteoarthritis or rheumatoid arthritis.

- **Arthroscopy:** In some cases, your doctor may refer you to a specialist for arthroscopy to see inside your joint. During arthroscopy, small incisions are made and a tiny camera is inserted to look inside your joint. The specialist watches a video screen to look for any abnormalities within your joint.

what is gout?

Gout is a type of arthritis caused by having high levels of uric acid in your bloodstream. It is thought to be caused by consuming too much protein, fat and alcohol. Too much uric acid causes crystals to form in your joints, which leads to pain and swelling. The pain can usually be eased by a short course of anti-inflammatory painkillers (see page 50).

will I need surgery?

The main complication that can result from severe osteoarthritis is joint replacement surgery. If the cartilage and bone become too damaged, your joints may become too painful or stiff to enable you to manage day-to-day activities. This is when a surgeon may become involved in your care and offer you a joint replacement. The most commonly replaced joints are the hip and knee. See page 53 for further information on joint replacement surgery and other surgical options.

rheumatoid arthritis

what is rheumatoid arthritis?

Rheumatoid arthritis (RA) is a serious disease. It is a chronic, progressive, auto-immune disease which is extremely painful, can cause severe disability, and ultimately affects a person's ability to carry out everyday tasks and their quality of life if it is undiagnosed or not treated effectively. RA can progress rapidly, but the speed of progression varies between individuals, and can cause swelling which damages the cartilage and bone around your joints. Any joint can be affected, but it is most commonly the hands, feet and wrists. It is a systemic disease, which means it can not only affect all the joints of the body but also the internal organs. This is not the case for everyone diagnosed with RA, but problems with the lungs, heart and eyes are all possible.

There are about 400,000 people in the UK with RA and overall it is the most common of the inflammatory diseases. In real terms about

12,000 people a year will develop RA. RA affects three times more women than men and onset is generally between 40 and 60 years of age, although you can get the disease at any age. There are around 12,000 children under the age of 16 with the juvenile form of the disease.

We're still not sure what causes RA. Unfortunately there is no cure, but much more is now understood about the inflammatory process associated with the disease and how it can be managed. This book aims to show you how with self-management you can help yourself, and minimize the impact of the disease on your quality of life.

The good news is that if you are diagnosed and treated early, your prognosis is significantly better than it was 20–30 years ago, thanks to research and the development of drugs which can modify the active disease process. Early diagnosis is critical, and research shows that a 3 month window of opportunity exists from onset of symptoms to starting treatment, which can prevent irreversible joint damage. Many people diagnosed now have a good quality of life in spite of having RA, and don't suffer the joint deformity that was once associated with the condition. Research also shows that in reality it can be up to a year between symptoms developing and the start of treatment. It is very important that people know how to recognise the symptoms and see their GP as soon as possible. GP education is also needed to ensure prompt referral for diagnosis and treatment.

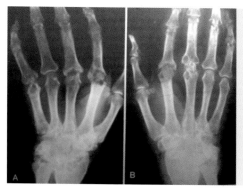

Figure 1.2 X-ray of the hands showing the deformity associated with RA

RA: the outlook
- The prognosis for people diagnosed with RA today is dramatically better than even 10 years ago.
- With early, aggressive treatment, you can lead a more normal life and limit joint damage.
- There are very effective new drugs available if conventional treatment does not work for you.
- Many new drugs are undergoing trials and more worldwide research is happening than ever before.
- Knowing about your disease will help you to come to terms with it and to make the right decisions about your treatment.

what causes RA?

People often ask, 'Why me?' Although the cause of rheumatoid arthritis is unknown, others in your family may have the condition too. It is not an inherited condition, but you can inherit a genetic predisposition to developing RA. Once you have developed rheumatoid arthritis it becomes a chronic disease and the body's own immune system attacks the lining of the joints.

signs and symptoms

Symptoms may include:

- joint swelling

- pain

- early morning joint stiffness

- poor sleep

- fatigue

- loss of weight

- flu-like symptoms

- unpredictable 'flare-ups' of inflammation.

If untreated the resulting disability may lead to loss of mobility, function and independence. Psychological effects such as depression and anxiety may also result.

how does RA differ from osteoarthritis?

The diagnosis of RA from the early symptoms can be very difficult. Joint swelling will be present in at least two joints, usually in the hands or feet. Along with this joint swelling, there is stiffness in the joints, particularly in the morning or after sitting for some time. This differs from osteoarthritis, which can also present with joint swelling and morning stiffness. But the morning stiffness in osteoarthritis usually only lasts 30 minutes, whereas in rheumatoid arthritis it is considerably longer. Patients with RA can also be woken in the night by joint pain and stiffness. This does not happen in osteoarthritis. Fatigue is

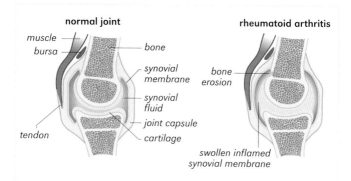

Figure 1.3 A normal knee joint compared to a knee joint with RA, showing the thinning of the cartilage and the inflamed synovial membrane which creates the swelling

pronounced in patients with RA and they may lose weight due to a poor appetite – again, this is not a feature of osteoarthritis.

how does RA damage joints?

We may not know much about what triggers RA, but we do know a lot about the inflammatory process that leads to joint damage. All medical treatments for RA are directed at suppressing or stopping parts of the joint-damaging process which is controlled by your immune system.

A normal joint is a complicated structure that allows movement. It has several parts, as shown in Figure 1.4.

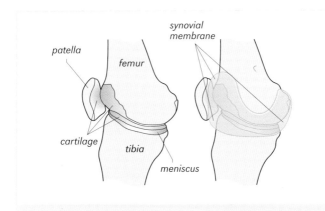

Figure 1.4 The components of the knee joint

Normal joints move painlessly, without you having to think about it. A joint needs adequate lubrication, just like the moving parts of an engine need oil. By understanding how a joint works it is easier to understand how it can go wrong. A joint is formed between two bones that move against each other. A good example is the knee. The ends of the bones in a joint are covered with smooth cartilage so that one surface can glide over the other. These gliding surfaces are within a 'joint capsule', which is a tough structure similar to a ligament, holding the joint together. The lining of the joint capsule is called the synovium or synovial membrane, and this structure produces the joint fluid that acts as a lubricant. The normal joint lining is thin; it has very few blood vessels and there are no white blood cells in it.

In the inflamed rheumatoid joint:

- The lining is very thick and is crowded with white blood cells that have entered it via new blood vessels in the thickened lining.

- These white blood cells produce a large number of chemical substances that cause inflammation.

- The joint becomes swollen, hot and tender to the touch, and function becomes a problem.

- Unchecked, this inflammatory process causes damage to the cartilage and bone in the joint.

- The inflamed synovial membrane creates inflammatory chemicals that eat into the bone and cartilage. The damage to the bone is seen in an X-ray as erosion.

- The chemicals produced by the white blood cells in the joint lining are released into the bloodstream and cause fatigue and general feelings of being unwell.

Suppression of inflammation in order to prevent long term joint damage is the goal of every rheumatologist, and the earlier and more aggressively someone with RA is treated, the better the long-term prognosis. Remission of RA is now being discussed as a possibility and if caught early enough, this is theoretically possible.

Other symptoms of RA
- dry or inflamed eyes
- fluid, fibrosis, or nodules (rare) in the lungs
- skin nodules and ulcers
- heart problems
- anaemia.

It's important to remember that not everyone gets all of these symptoms, and some are more common than others. Symptoms that affect the heart and lungs are less common, so you should not worry that they will affect you. The sooner you are diagnosed and see a rheumatologist, the sooner you can start the treatment which can prevent many of these symptoms from ever developing.

how are RA and OA managed?

specialist help

Along with the medication you may need to take, there are many people who can help you to manage your RA or OA. It is unlikely that you will need the services of all these professionals at once, but it is essential to know who they are and how to access them when you need them. It's a good idea to keep all the phone numbers close at hand so you can find them as soon as you need them. Treatment makes an important difference to the symptoms of inflammation and damage to the joints for those with RA, and the ability to cope with arthritis in general.

- **The rheumatologist** will diagnose and manage your RA. He/she will request any tests that you need to diagnose and monitor your condition, prescribe medication and monitor how this controls your RA.

- **The nurse practitioner** works closely with the rheumatologist and will monitor you between visits to the specialist. He/she is one of the most important people for you to know and will often be key in providing support and teaching you about RA. They will also be able to arrange investigations and discuss any findings with your doctor to make sure you are getting the best care. In most units they also operate a nurse-led helpline.

- **The physiotherapist** provides important non-drug treatments for both osteoarthritis and RA, including exercise, acupuncture, and pain-relieving strategies that you can also use at home. Working with a physiotherapist will allow you to develop, maintain and restore movement and function during and after a flare-up of RA. If you have OA your physiotherapist will help you strengthen your joints and improve your self management and overall function.

- **The occupational therapist** works closely with you to provide resting and support splints for painful joints, and equipment to make day-to-day tasks easier. Resting splints are more commonly used for people with RA. Occupational therapists focus on helping people with arthritis to achieve independence in all areas of their lives in spite of their joint pain. They are really helpful in assessing your work place to make sure you can stay at work when you have RA. They work closely with physiotherapists to support overall treatment.

- **The podiatrist** studies and treats disorders of the foot, ankle and leg. Podiatrists work closely with physiotherapists in the management of arthritis and are the experts in biomechanical assessment, which involves looking at the posture and movement of your feet. They will prescribe custom-made insoles (orthotics) if you need help to control your foot position as a result of pain or joint damage. This can have a great impact on pain prevention and muscle imbalance.

- **Pain management clinics** have specialist doctors, nurses and physiotherapists who understand chronic pain and only work in this area. Your doctor may refer you if your pain is difficult to control. These clinics can prescribe drugs to manage your pain and also offer cognitive behavioural therapy (CBT) which can be a great help in managing chronic pain (see page 46).

- **The pharmacist** is the best person to advise you on which medications can help you without a prescription. Use the same pharmacist for all your prescription and non-prescription drugs, as they can then monitor what you take and check for any unwanted interactions between different drugs.

- **Counsellers** can be really useful in helping you come to terms with the emotional difficulties of living with RA. Your GP can refer you to see someone who is best placed to help you (see page 48 for self-help advice).

- **NHS Direct** is a useful source of advice if you are concerned and unable to see your physiotherapist or GP. It can help you decide on the most appropriate management for your condition, and advise you who you should see if things become worse. The number for NHS Direct is 0845 46 47.

- **The dietician** can recommend foods to boost your immune system, or ensure your vitamin and mineral intake is maintained so that medication and reduced activity during a flare-up do not have too great an impact on your health. Most people would benefit from dietary advice, but as an arthritis sufferer it is easy to gain weight, as exercise may be limited when you are in pain. Simple advice can have a major impact on your weight and subsequently your pain.

- **The orthopaedic surgeon** has a role in the management of arthritis if all other measures have failed. Your doctor will refer you to a surgeon if necessary. Surgery to deal with structural change can be used if the joint becomes damaged, and this will aim to reduce pain and improve your function and independence. This is not always as large scale as a joint replacement. Small procedures can be performed with the use of a small camera (arthroscopy) which can be very helpful in reducing pain and improving movement in a joint.

- **Voluntary organisations** such as NRAS, ARC and AC offer support and information. Find their contact details in the back of this book.

effective medication

Effective and early treatment of RA makes a big impact on the course of the disease by improving quality of life, preventing joint damage and reducing the need for surgery. Treatment should, in an ideal world, begin within three months of the onset of symptoms, so seeing your doctor as soon as possible is important. Getting a diagnosis can sometimes take a lot longer than six months, depending on your symptoms and how they affect you. If the initial course of medication does not help to reduce your symptoms, then it should be changed as soon as possible to prevent irreversible joint damage. It can sometimes take more than one attempt to find the most effective medication for you, but this is part and parcel of having and managing RA.

Your doctor can prescribe different kinds of drugs, both to suppress the inflammation and to prevent the joint damage caused by the disease process. The drugs used to treat RA fit into four main categories:

- painkillers and non-steroidal anti-inflammatory drugs (NSAIDs)

- disease modifying anti-rheumatoid drugs (DMARDs)

- steroids (tablets and injections)

- biologic agents (given directly into the bloodstream in a drip).

It is known that DMARDs and biologic treatments slow down or even stop joint damage. NICE (National Institute for Health and Clinical Excellence) are advocating multiple therapy at the onset of RA to improve outcome and limit joint damage. See pages 51–52 to find out more about these drugs and what they do.

Research is constantly producing new treatments for RA, and you can keep in touch with all new developments and research on the National Rheumatoid Arthritis Society (NRAS) website (www.rheumatoid. org.uk).

The good news is that effective treatments for RA are reducing the need for surgery. Many rheumatology centres are now reporting that the number of patients needing orthopaedic surgery over the last 10 to 15 years has significantly declined.

when to see your doctor

● The golden rule is that if you have swelling of more than two joints and stiffness in the joints in the mornings for longer than half an hour, you should go and see your doctor.

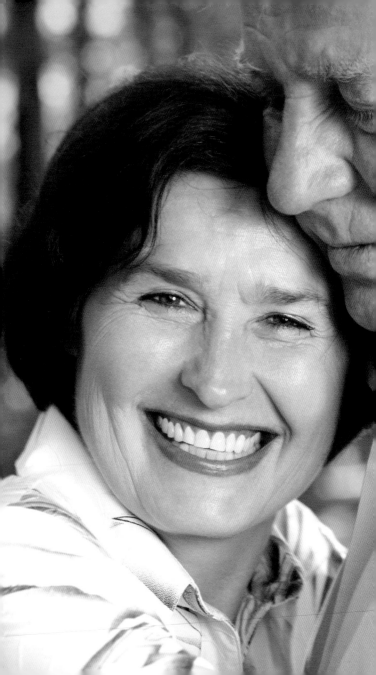

part 2
helping yourself to health

where do I start?

The first thing to think about is what you can do to help yourself. If you take an active role in managing your arthritis with your doctor and health care team, this will help you feel that you are in charge of your disease, rather than vice versa. Studies have shown that people who take control of their treatment and actively manage their arthritis experience less pain and function better.

Self management skills:

- Setting goals and action plans

- Getting the most from your medication

- Managing stress and your emotions

- Pacing your daily activities

- Finding healthcare resources in the community

- Understanding the importance of exercise, healthy eating and stopping smoking

- Manage fatigue (especially if you have RA).

To help you do this, this part of the book begins with an MOT questionnaire below. This will help you think about what you can change to improve your health and manage your condition. This is followed by advice on various self-help strategies for how to manage your arthritis, including how to treat yourself when you have a flare-up, how to pace yourself to avoid flare-ups, and how to improve your general health and fitness by eating healthily and stopping smoking. The rest of part 2 is designed to help you find out what kind of help you can get, and where to get it, such as physiotherapy and cognitive behavioural therapy, and finally gives advice on what prescription medications or other treatments are available.

making a start
Take a long hard look at the unhealthy aspects of your lifestyle and be honest with yourself. Choose one thing that you know needs to change to have a positive impact on your health. You may decide that you don't eat enough vegetables, get enough exercise or take your medication the way you should.

Once you decide what you want to change, think about how to make things happen. Write down a specific goal – the more specific you are with your goal, the more likely you are to succeed. Instead of saying, 'I'm going to do more exercise,' decide what kind of exercise you will do, on which days and at what time you will exercise. Your new goal could be: 'After work on Monday, Wednesday and Friday, I will walk for 30 minutes in the park.' Just make sure you plan ahead.

your personal MOT
Even if you have had arthritis for many years, it's worth thinking about where you have come from and to judge what impact this may have on your current health and fitness. If you have been newly diagnosed with arthritis, then you definitely need to give some thought to your exercise

history so that you can start or continue to exercise and avoid aggravating your symptoms.

The questions below are designed to give you a brief MOT. The questionnaire is not designed to give you a full medical check-up – only a professional can do that, so visit your GP or a physiotherapist if you are significantly overweight, unable to control your joint pain or have other ongoing medical problems. Your MOT will help you to focus on the 'here and now' – looking at your general health and your arthritic pain, spotting the tell-tale signs of potential problems that may be lurking just around the corner. Answer the questions as honestly as you can and then count how many 'yes' and 'no' answers you have.

MOT questionnaire	yes	no
1 Would you describe yourself as unfit?		
2 Would you describe yourself as overweight?		
3 Are you off work because of your arthritis?		
4 Are you worried about exercising in case it makes your pain worse?		
5 Are you worried or not happy about taking medication for your pain?		
6 Does your pain affect your mood and make you feel frustrated or depressed?		
7 Have you had pain for many years?		
8 Do you have hot swollen joints at the moment that you have not seen your doctor about?		
9 Could your diet be healthier or more varied?		
10 Do you smoke or have you ever smoked?		
11 Have your joints become more painful recently, along with other symptoms of feeling unwell?		

The more 'yes' answers you have, the more things you can change to have a positive effect on your health and your arthritis. If you answered 'yes' to either question 8 or 11 you may benefit from treatment, and need to seek advice to make sure you are doing all you can to manage your arthritis. This is explained in more detail below. It is likely that your fitness will have been directly affected by your arthritis, and recognising this is the first step to making the changes that will improve your health and your quality of life.

yes to questions 1 and 2:

If you think you are unfit and overweight, then you probably are! To be honest, most people have periods in their life when this is the case whether they have arthritis or not. Arthritis does make it harder to exercise but not impossible, and once you make a start it will help you manage your pain better and lose weight too. There is plenty of medical evidence that losing weight will help improve your joint pain. Part 3 includes exercises which will both ease your joint pain and gently get you back to fitness.

weight check

Take a look at Figure 2.1 and find your height at the side and your weight along the top or bottom. Follow a line across the chart from your height until you reach the line that corresponds with your weight. Are you the right weight for your height? If not, it is time to do something about it – even small changes to your lifestyle can help you lose weight. See the healthy eating advice on page 39 and the easy-to-follow exercise programme on pages 69–76.

yes to question 3:

If you are off work as a result of your arthritis, it is important to think about returning as soon as you can. If your pain is severe and limiting your movement, then it is important to have a few days off to allow your joints to settle and get any swelling under control. You may need to see

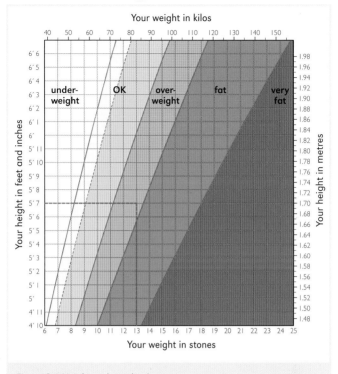

Figure 2.1 Height and weight chart

your GP if you have OA for a change of medication, but try over-the-counter painkillers too. If you have RA you will need to contact your consultant or nurse specialist – they can refer you for physiotherapy if needed. If you have OA and need treatment from a physiotherapist you can arrange this privately or your GP can refer you on the NHS.

Research has shown that people who are off work for six months or more as a result of a chronic condition are less likely to return to work. This is not just because of pain and loss of fitness, but also the psychological issues that can arise when you have chronic pain. Many of these problems can be addressed with advice, reassurance and knowing all the facts about pain.

> **TIP**
>
> 'When my knees hurt I walk down stairs backwards. It doesn't hurt as much – my physio says it's because I'm using my muscles differently.'
>
> John, OA, Scotland

yes to question 4:

It is very normal to worry, and when you are in pain it is difficult to think of anything that will help, least of all exercise. The benefits of exercise for arthritis have been known for many years, but the important thing is to pace yourself and do the right exercises for your level of pain and fitness. Part 3 includes exercises that you can use even when you are in severe pain and will teach you how to progress to the more active exercises when you feel ready.

There are many myths about pain which can be unhelpful and stop you getting better. Use this book to make sure you understand as much as you can about your arthritis, and read especially about the importance of pacing yourself (page 36) and how you might benefit from cognitive behavioural therapy (page 46).

yes to question 5:

It is important to take painkillers, DMARDs (see page 51) or steroids if you need them, as this will help you move more freely and get better more quickly. By taking medication regularly instead of waiting for pain to increase, you will help keep pain at bay. If your drugs control your pain and allow you to exercise, this has the added advantage of enabling you to strengthen your joints, which helps to reduce pain, which in turn allows you to take less medication.

Many people don't like taking medication because of worries about addiction or side-effects, but it is an essential part of managing your symptoms, especially if you have RA. The risks of becoming addicted are actually very small if you are taking tablets correctly and for the right reasons. Side-effects are possible, but there are many different drugs available, and if some don't agree with you or don't relieve your pain, chat to your consultant, GP or pharmacist about what else is available. On page 50 you will find more about the different types of drugs available for both osteoarthritis and RA.

yes to question 6:

Many people find that they feel low or frustrated when they are in pain. Be reassured that this is a perfectly normal response to having pain and not being able to do the things you would like to take for granted. If you have had arthritis and pain for a long time and think that you may be depressed, it is important not to ignore this. Treating your mental health and well-being is a big part of treating your arthritis. Confide in your GP, who will be able to talk you through the options that will help. You may choose anti-depressants, counselling or both. Improving your mood will definitely reduce the pain you are feeling. Your pain and your mood are very closely linked to chemical changes in your body and taking drugs to help your pain or mood helps to bring these chemicals back into balance.

yes to question 7:

If you have had OA or RA for many years, you may feel that nothing has helped or can help you. The truth is there is no cure for chronic pain, but surgery is an option for some people with severe joint pain caused by both forms of arthritis. Surgery is not an easy option, but it can improve your function, mobility and reduce your joint pain. If you have RA and your pain is not under control you should have your treatment and medication reviewed. It is normal to have ups and downs, when your pain is sometimes better controlled than others. However, the good news is that you can make the good times last longer and have less severe flare ups if you exercise to improve your overall fitness, take the medication you need and make a few lifestyle changes that will impact on your overall health. Read the advice on pacing (page 36) and CBT (page 46), and then give the exercises in part 3 a go.

yes to question 8:

If you have hot and swollen joints that are not settling with the use of ice, rest and your usual medication, its time to get things checked out.

If you have RA, it may also be a sign that your condition is not being managed by the medication you are taking. You may need an injection of steroids into the joint to help things settle down. Have it checked out by your consultant or nurse specialist team, who if necessary will be able to do this for you or will send you to someone who can.

yes to question 9:
A healthy and balanced diet is so important for good health and maintaining a healthy weight. If you answered 'yes', take a look at the healthy eating advice on page 39.

yes to question 10:
If you smoke, now is the time to stop. There are 2000 deaths every week in the UK as a result of smoking-related diseases. Smoking is a direct cause of peripheral vascular disease (narrowing of your arteries) which causes bad circulation. If you have RA you are at a greater risk of developing this and there is research to show that smoking will make your RA worse. Poor circulation will slow down your ability to heal after a flare-up of your pain. See page 42 for information on stopping smoking.

yes to question 11:
If you are having more pain, or are feeling unwell and have swelling in your joints, you should see your GP or if you have RA your usual management team. This could be a sign that things needs investigating for either condition and you may need some tests, or may just need different painkillers or anti-inflammatories that will help.

Now you know your MOT results and what you need to think about, it is time to find out how you can make the lifestyle changes to improve your health and your arthritis for the better.

managing a flare-up

Even though the management of osteoarthritis and RA are very different, there are some things that you can do that will help both forms of arthritis: these are general things you can change that will help many aspects of your health, such as losing weight, changing your diet or controlling stress. Experience will tell you what happens to you during a flare-up, and you may need to increase your medication, manage your emotional health better, use ice, or rest. Below I will run through all these aspects of self-management, but it is up to you to implement the changes. They are not all quick fixes for use in times of flare-ups, but many are lifestyle choices that will influence how severe those flare-ups can be. If these actions don't help, you may need to seek further advice, especially if your symptoms start to impact on your daily activities or you feel your arthritis is not being controlled by your medication.

P.R.I.C.E.

If you are experiencing pain or inflammation in your joint, use the P.R.I.C.E method outlined below for 12 to 24 hours. Reduce your activities so you don't use the joint repeatedly. Take a 10 minute break every hour – for example, when you're at work take a break from sitting at your desk.

- **Protect:** stop the activity to avoid further damage to the joint.

- **Rest:** this will prevent further damage and allow you to elevate your legs if your knees and ankles hurt, to reduce pressure and inflammation.

- **Ice** will reduce the swelling. It should be applied for no more than 10 minutes, directly to the joint. Any longer may result in an ice burn and damage tissue further. A cold pack or plastic bag filled with crushed ice and wrapped in a wet towel will help avoid an ice burn. You can buy gel packs to keep in the freezer, although my patients tell me bags of frozen peas are just as good! Apply ice four to eight times a day. Don't use cold treatments if you have poor circulation or numbness.

- **Compression** will help keep swelling to a minimum. Compression bandages such as tubi-grip are the easiest to apply, but splints are also available – ask your doctor or physiotherapist. If your ankles are swollen, flight socks and compression tights are really helpful. Some chemists sell all these items.

- **Elevation:** keep the joint elevated to reduce blood flow and swelling to the area.

Both heat and cold can relieve pain in your joints. Heat relieves stiffness, and cold can relieve muscle spasms. Many people with osteoarthritis or RA find painful joints benefit from using a heat pad, hot water bottle or warm bath. This is not always helpful if your RA is going through a flare-up and ice is more helpful. Heat should be warm, not hot, and can be applied for 20 minutes several times a day. If you are having a flare-up, cool the pain of swollen, hot joints with ice packs.

> **TIP**
> 'You can make re-usable ice packs from ice-cube bags and jelly. Melt the jelly as you would normally, pour it into the ice-cube bags and allow it to set. You can keep these in the freezer so you always have an ice pack ready for use.'
>
> Mavis, RA, Yorkshire

Creams and gels available from your pharmacist may provide temporary relief from arthritic pain caused by OA. Some creams reduce the pain by creating a hot or cool sensation. Other creams contain medication that is absorbed into your skin. Ask your pharmacist for advice on which is best suited for you and the other drugs you are taking. Pain creams work best on joints that are close to the surface of your skin, such as your knees and fingers. If you have RA check with your management team before trying new drugs or creams.

exercise

Regular exercise is the way forward, and part 3 will show you what you can do safely. By sticking to gentle exercises, such as walking or swimming, you can protect your joints while increasing your endurance and strengthening the muscles around your joint. This will make your joint more stable and help to minimise your pain. It is common sense to rest tender, injured or swollen joints, but not forever. If you feel new joint pain, stop. New pain that lasts more than two hours after you exercise probably means you've overdone it. Once you learn how your body responds to exercise, you can push yourself further while still pacing yourself (see page 36).

flare-ups and exercise

If you have had RA for a while, the likelihood is that you will have had a flare-up of some sort. A history of flare-ups places you at a higher risk of joint stiffness, problems with the surfaces of your joints, and muscle wasting and weakness. This is mainly due to the effect of inflammation in the joints if not brought under control, and is more of a problem if you have RA.

Insufficient exercise and a lack of strength and conditioning will make you weaker and can make pain much worse. Incorporating exercise into your life will help you to reduce the impact of a flare-up. Part 3 contains recommended exercises for each area of the body and suggestions for the best exercises to try when you are in severe pain (see page 88).

Having successfully advised and treated many people over the years to achieve pain management, I can't stress enough how important it is for you to persevere with the professional advice and exercise programmes prescribed. When pain comes back after a period of better management, it's usually because people haven't been keeping up their exercise programme.

lose weight

Being overweight increases the stress on your weight-bearing joints – your knees, hips and ankles. Excess body fat has been linked to an increase in inflammation, so weight management is advisable for this reason too. Even losing a small amount of weight can relieve pressure on your joints and reduce pain. Aim to lose 0.5–1 kg (1–2 pounds) a week at most. Your doctor can refer you to a dietician if you need help to lose weight, but most people find that by making small changes to their diet and by increasing the amount of exercise, weight loss happens. A healthy diet can help you control your weight and maintain your overall health, allowing you to deal better with your arthritis. However, there is no special diet for treating arthritis, and although there is a huge amount of dietary advice aimed at people with arthritis, there is no research to suggest that eating any particular food will make your joint pain or inflammation better or worse. Read through the diet advice on page 39, which summarises that given by the National Rheumatoid Arthritis Society, and see the Society's website (rheumatoid.org.uk) for more information.

Little or no exercise will greatly increase the risk of weight gain if what you are eating is not modified when you are unable to exercise. If you can't exercise because of a flare-up of your symptoms, try keeping a diet diary for a week or two to help spot where unnecessary snacks could be cut out.

avoid stressing your joints

There is always more than one way to do anything, and there is always a way to complete your normal day with reduced stress on your joints. An occupational therapist can help you discover ways to do everyday tasks without putting extra stress on your already painful joint. For instance, a toothbrush with a large grip could make brushing your teeth easier if you have osteoarthritis or RA in your fingers. You can modify any handle with pipe lagging or foam to make it wider and easier to hold. A special seat in your shower could help relieve the pain of standing if you have osteoarthritis in your knees. It is also easy to make simple changes at work to your workstation that can make things easier for you.

HINTS AND TIPS

I have learnt many tips from my patients over the years, and I have listed some here and in the tip boxes throughout the book.

- Tights – cut off the toes and wear these when going to the chiropodist so there is no need to undress.
- Long handled shoe horns and elastic or coiled laces that don't have to be tied help when putting on shoes, boots or trainers.
- Use a wooden spatula for lifting up a bra strap.
- Use fitted sheets that do not require tucking in. Use a large wooden spoon or spatula to lever the last two corners over the mattress. Start with the corners that are least accessible or most difficult.
- Use smaller, lightweight towels and face flannels to dry yourself as they are much easier to handle.

The resting splints of the past are still available, but there are many more functional options available now that are not bulky and will support your joints without limiting you too much. These can be helpful to use during the day when you are at work. Your physiotherapist or occupational therapist can advise you before you buy and also show you what is available.

Other ways you can reduce stress on your joints are:

- **Get a helping hand:** Splints and adaptive devices can help reduce stress on your painful joint. Gripping and grabbing tools may make it easier to work in the kitchen if your fingers are affected. Look in catalogues and medical supply shops for ideas (see box).

- **Spread the load:** Use both hands to lift a heavy pan. Try using a walking stick to take weight off your knee or hip as you walk. Slipping some foam pipe lagging under the handles makes carrying heavy shopping bags easier on the small joints in your hands. This is available from most DIY shops.

- **Check your posture:** Poor posture causes uneven weight distribution and may strain ligaments and muscles. The easiest way to improve your posture is to be aware of how you sit and stand. Relax your muscles, and use a mirror to help you see if you are standing evenly. Make sure you stand with equal weight on both legs, and when you sit make sure you are well supported, instead of slumping or using a chair with no back rest. Think about your sleeping posture too. If you can, invest in a good mattress and pillow. See below for advice.

- **Use your strongest muscles:** Don't push open a heavy door with your hand – lean into it. To pick up an object, bend your knees and squat while keeping your back straight.

- **Choose the right shoes:** Wearing comfortable shoes that properly support your weight is especially important if you have arthritis in your weight-bearing joints or back. Gel insoles are also helpful to reduce the weight and pressure on the small joints in the feet.

finding equipment
These websites are great places to get equipment that will help you with day-to-day tasks. But before you spend a fortune, speak to an occupational therapist who can advise you on the things that can help you the most. Some suppliers have shops or showrooms where you can try before you buy – your occupational therapist or social services should be able to direct you to the nearest one.

www.aidstomobility.org
www.help-my-mobility.co.uk
www.physiosupplies.co.uk
www.physiomed.co.uk

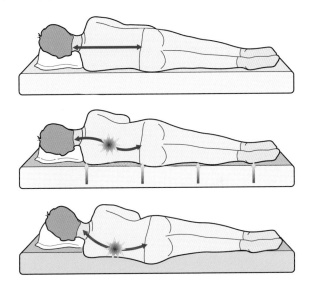

Figure 2.2 Good sleeping posture (top)

TIP

'I use pipe lagging to help me carry shopping bags. Holding the foam lagging in your hand and placing the bag handles through the split in the foam stops the plastic handles digging in and making my fingers swell. You can also use it on gardening tools, kitchen knives and resistance bands for your exercises.'

Barbara, RA, London

● avoiding flare-ups: pacing yourself

Pacing yourself is one of the most important concepts to practice when you have arthritis, and will help you stop doing either too much or too little, both of which are very common. Here are two common scenarios which you may recognise.

- **Overdoing it**
  You are not in pain, so you run around getting all the jobs done that you haven't been able to do because of a previous flare-up. Because you feel good, you keep going, happily ticking things off your list. As you carry on you feel increasing pain until you can't keep it up and you have to rest. Unfortunately the pain is worse after your rest and worse still the next day, sometimes for two or three days. As the cycle continues, you have to rest for longer periods, putting you off doing the activity again. You lose fitness, and become frustrated and depressed.

- **Underdoing it**
  You are in pain and only get relief when you rest. You have had to stop working as a result of your pain and now spend much of your time resting, unable to go out or to the gym as a result of your pain. Your family are supportive, and do your shopping for you or run errands. You have become unfit and have put on weight, but can't do anything about it because of your pain. You may lose confidence, start to feel that you don't have a role within the workplace or family, and may feel depressed and have difficulty sleeping.

Both of these are common ways in which people try to manage their arthritis. Unfortunately, neither is effective and in the long run the pain and disability increase. Learning how to pace yourself can be hard, but if you follow these four easy steps you will be able to use the pacing principle in all areas of your life.

step 1: measure your activity

You probably have very little idea how long it takes you to perform various tasks before you start to experience pain. For you to control your pain, you need to know how long you can continue with a certain job or activity before your pain will increase. The key to this is to time yourself and work out how many minutes it takes to bring on your pain.

step 2: set yourself a limit

To set yourself a limit, take the time you measured and take off 20 per cent. This is your limit. For example, if your pain comes on after 10 minutes of ironing your limit is 8 minutes. You must not go over your limit: use a timer to make you stop.

step 3: stick to the limit you set

This is the hard bit – when the timer says stop, go and do something else or rest. For how long? That is for you to decide – it may vary from a few minutes if you have been ironing to a few days if you were gardening. The idea is to find your happy medium. It may be frustrating but I guarantee it will work.

step 4: increase your limit

One you know your limit and you can stick to it and get the job done without increasing your pain, it is time to increase your limit. Be careful by how much you increase your limit and decide before you start how much more time you will allow. Jumping from 8 minutes of housework to 30 minutes is likely to be too much too soon – 15 minutes may be more realistic and keep you active and pain free.

In time you will see an increase in what you are able to do without knocking yourself out. It often helps to keep a record of how you are increasing your activities – you will be able to look back and see how far you have come.

use pacing to increase:
- how long you can spend doing housework
- how long you can spend gardening
- how long you can stay at work when you first go back
- how many days a week you can work when you first go back
- how long you can exercise or how many exercises you can do
- how long you can drive for before you need to get out and stretch.

All the decisions you make will have short and long term benefits. By considering both the pros and cons of each option, in terms of benefits now and later, you will be able to make a more informed choice. For example, the house or car may need cleaning, but you are going to a wedding tomorrow which will be more active than your normal day. Take the car to the car wash so you have a clean car for the wedding and consider getting a cleaner. If getting a cleaner is not an option for you, leave the cleaning for a few days. You may have a messy house, but at least you will enjoy the wedding!

Finally, remember to rest when you are tired. RA in particular can make you prone to fatigue and muscle weakness. If you feel exhausted it makes everything you do an effort. An hour's rest or short nap that doesn't interfere with your night-time sleep may help.

TIP

'So I can keep hold of my soap I put the bar inside an old pop sock. I can still get it to lather but it's not as slippery and easier to pick up if you do drop it.'

Shirley, RA, London

● self-help: healthy eating

You will have worked out from the MOT questionnaire that healthy eating is a key part of having a healthy lifestyle and managing your arthritis. Eating healthily is not as hard as you may think and the benefits are well worth the effort.

If you are not eating a healthy balanced diet, you will soon start to feel the effects and will notice these even more as you start to exercise. Imagine driving a car: you wouldn't dream of setting off on a journey without enough fuel. A healthy diet also helps to maintain a normal body weight and can reduce your risk of developing heart disease, high blood pressure and high cholesterol. This is why you need to be aware of what kinds of food you are putting into your body, not just to feed yourself but also as a way of keeping yourself healthy.

Drinking is just as important as eating. Most people don't drink enough day-to-day and therefore function at a level of dehydration. If you feel thirsty, it's already too late: you are dehydrated. Your body

what is a healthy diet?
A healthy diet contains:

- plenty of carbohydrates or starchy foods like bread, rice, pasta, breakfast cereals, potatoes, and sweet potatoes – look for higher fibre versions where possible (like wholemeal bread or pasta)
- at least five portions of a variety of fruit and vegetables daily
- moderate amounts of dairy products (or alternatives if you don't tolerate them) – look for low fat versions where possible
- moderate amount of protein, which is found in meat, fish, eggs, beans, and lentils
- the occasional treat (foods that are higher in fat, salt or added sugar should only be eaten in moderation)
- minimal salt – always read the label.

needs 2–2.5 litres of fluid a day and when you exercise you will need more. The easiest way to check how hydrated you are is to monitor the colour of your urine. It should be a pale straw colour – any darker and you're already dehydrated.

Healthy eating need not be expensive – if you cook meals that use starchy foods and fruit and vegetables, aiming to eat less fat, salt and added sugar, it can actually work out much cheaper.

Whole grain, high fibre foods tend to release their energy more slowly so you feel full for longer and are less likely to snack on fatty and sugary foods. Fruit and vegetables provide you with fibre that keeps your bowel healthy and also help you feel full. Figure 2.3 shows you the different food groups and how much of each should make up your daily meals.

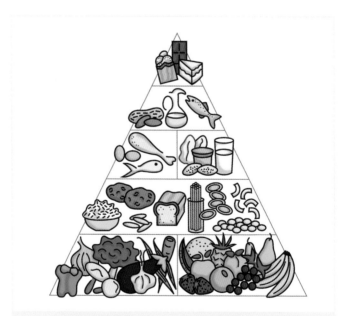

Figure 2.3 Balancing the food groups for a healthy diet

Good quantities of fresh fruit and vegetables are the way forward. Heavily processed or pre-packaged food is not only generally high in sugar but also high in salt and fat, all of which can contribute to weight problems, raise your cholesterol and raise your blood pressure. All of these factors will make managing your health harder.

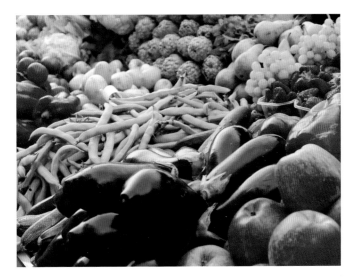

fish oils and omega-3 fatty acids

There is some evidence to show that omega-3 fats, taken as vitamin supplements, can improve the symptoms of both RA and osteoarthritis, but research shows they have to be taken in very high doses. Omega-3 fatty acids are found in oily fish like mackerel, sardines, herring, salmon, trout and fresh tuna. Eating oily fish two or three times a week can provide you with a good amount of omega-3. If you are not a fan of eating fish, taking fish oil supplements can easily increase the amounts of omega-3 in your diet.

Apart from fish oils (see box), there is little evidence that vitamin supplements are of specific benefit if you have RA or osteoarthritis. Some supplements are reported anecdotally to work for some people, and that is fine for them as long as money is not being spent on unproven supplements. However, the best way to get your quota of vitamins is to eat a healthy, balanced diet.

If you are planning to make a change to your diet, it is always advisable to have an assessment by a registered dietician. If you want more help and advice on losing weight there are many options: you can join a slimming club, ask your GP to refer you to a dietician, or get advice online from the government-funded Eatwell campaign. Some useful websites are:

www.the-gi-diet.org
www.eatwell.gov.uk
www.weightwatchers.co.uk
www.dietchef.co.uk
www.slimmingworld.com

self-help: stopping smoking

One of the greatest ways to have a positive impact on your health is to stop smoking. You may be wondering what stopping smoking has to do with your arthritis. However, smoking affects your general health and your circulation, and this has a direct impact on how quickly you heal and recover from injury and pain. If you have RA or osteoarthritis you really should stop smoking for the good of both your overall health and your joints. There is strong research evidence that shows RA is more severe in smokers.

Smoking causes numerous diseases and health problems, and not just for the smoker. Both smokers and non-smokers develop smoking-related disease. For this reason, smoking is now banned in public places and a wide range of support services has been developed to help you quit smoking.

reasons to quit

You may want to give up smoking for many reasons, from wanting to improve your health, to saving money or reducing potential harm to your family. In the UK one person dies from a smoking-related disease every four minutes. Smoking places you at a greater risk of developing heart disease, high blood pressure and peripheral vascular disease (PVD). These are some of the other diseases caused by smoking:

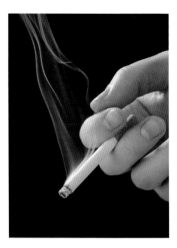

- lung cancer (smoking causes over 80 per cent of all lung cancer deaths)

- heart disease

- bronchitis

- strokes

- stomach ulcers

- leukaemia

- gangrene

- other cancers e.g. mouth and throat cancer.

Smoking can also make having a cold, chest problems and allergies like hay fever much worse, as well as increasing the number of wrinkles on your face and causing bad breath. It can make you cough and feel short of breath when you exercise.

As well as improving your own health dramatically, here are some of the other advantages of stopping smoking:

- **It will boost your sex appeal:** it's a myth that smoking helps you lose weight – in fact it can cause cellulite. And kissing someone with a mouth like an ashtray is just revolting.

- **It will improve your sense of taste and smell** – a perfect side effect for enjoying your healthy new diet!

- **You will save money:** calculate how much you spend on cigarettes each week and multiply this by 52. Work out just how much smoking is costing you every year and you might be surprised how much you could save or what you could buy instead.

- **You will protect your family's health:** breathing in other people's cigarette smoke can also cause cancer. Children exposed to second-hand smoke are twice as likely to get chest problems and more likely to get ear and throat infections and asthma, while smoking during pregnancy can affect your baby's health as well as your own.

types of treatment

When willpower alone is not enough, there are various treatments and plenty of support services to help you kick the habit. Many chemists offer a 'stop smoking' service and can advise you on the products available to help you quit. There are many types of nicotine replacement therapy treatments, delivering nicotine in various ways, including gum, patches, microtabs (which dissolve under the tongue), lozenges, inhalators and nasal sprays. Other drugs that can help you to stop smoking are Zyban (bupropion hydrochloride), which changes the way that your body responds to nicotine, and Champix (varenicline), which works by reducing your craving for a cigarette and by reducing the effects you feel if you do have a cigarette. Both these treatments are only available on prescription and cannot be used if you are pregnant.

helpful contacts

Smokers are four times more likely to quit by using the NHS Stop Smoking Services together with nicotine replacement therapy, than they are by using willpower alone. Find your nearest NHS service by:

- visiting the NHS Smokefree website (http://smokefree.nhs.uk) for England and Wales, or Smokeline (www.clearingtheairscotland.com) in Scotland

- texting GIVE UP and your full postcode to 88088

- telephoning the NHS Smoking Helpline (0800 022 4332) in England and Wales, or Smokeline (0800 84 84 84) in Scotland

- asking your GP or pharmacist.

The NHS Smoking Helpline in England and Wales offers free practical advice about giving up smoking, as well as a free information pack, while in Scotland, Smokeline provides free confidential advice and support. Both Smokefree and Smokeline offer an 'Ask an Expert' service.

getting help

A big part of self-management is knowing when to ask for help when you need it. This support can come from friends and family, as well as from your doctor, a support group, or someone else with your condition. Some of the types of help, from therapies to drug treatment, are described below.

physiotherapy

Ask your doctor for a referral to a physiotherapist if you want help to get started. A physiotherapist can work with you to create an individualised exercise plan to strengthen the muscles around your joints, increase the range of motion in your joints and reduce your pain. This is very important if you have RA as working with a physiotherapist will make sure you pace yourself and protect your

TIP

'My easy-reach was one of the best things I ever bought. It just makes reaching to pick things up easy. I didn't want one at first because I thought I was too young to have things like that. But it really made a big difference to my life.'

Ken, OA, Yorkshire

joints. This may be the confidence boost you need to start the self-management advice in this book.

chronic pain classes

Some hospitals and centres run classes for people with osteoarthritis or chronic pain. Ask your doctor or physiotherapist about classes in your area or check with Arthritis Care (www.arthritiscare.org.uk) or the Arthritis Research Campaign (www.arc.org.uk). These classes teach skills that help you manage your pain, and you will also meet other people with your condition and learn their tips for reducing joint pain or coping with pain.

cognitive behavioural therapy (CBT)

Medications and other treatments may be a key part of managing your arthritis and the associated pain, but successful treatment depends just as much on your attitude and your emotional health. Your ability to cope despite pain often determines how much of an impact your condition will have on your day-to-day life. Studies show that people who take control of their pain treatment and actively manage their arthritis experience less pain and function better.

CBT is a way of talking about how you think about yourself, how you relate to the world, and how what you do affects your thoughts and feelings. In relation to your arthritis, it can help you focus on the problems and difficulties you are having, instead of on the causes of your distress or symptoms. One of the ways it works is by breaking problems down into smaller parts, making it easier to see how many things – your thoughts, emotions, physical feelings and actions – relate to your arthritis. All these things are closely linked, and how you think about your condition can affect how you feel physically and emotionally.

There are helpful and unhelpful ways of reacting to most situations, depending on how you think about them, and when we are distressed, in pain, or both, we are more likely to jump to conclusions and to see things in unhelpful ways. It is easy for a vicious circle to set in (fig. 2.4). CBT can help you to break this vicious circle of unhelpful thinking, feelings and behaviour. When you see how these interactions can influence how you behave, you can change them, and this includes what you do about your arthritis.

CBT can be done individually, in a group, or even by using a self-help book. If you see a therapist, you will usually have sessions lasting between 30 and 60 minutes, and after discussing your past life events and background will agree on short-, medium- and long-term goals. Over the period of treatment – probably between six weeks and six months – you will look at your thoughts, feelings and behaviours to work out whether they are unrealistic or unhelpful, how they interact and how they affect you. The therapist will then help you to work out how to change unhelpful thoughts and behaviours.

The availability of CBT varies between different areas and there may be a waiting list for treatment. Your GP can refer you. The beauty of CBT is that you can continue to develop your skills by yourself even after your sessions have finished.

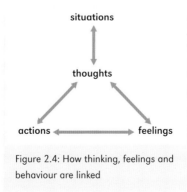

Figure 2.4: How thinking, feelings and behaviour are linked

information on CBT

For further information see the CBT web pages of PsychNet-UK (www.psychnet-uk.com/psychotherapy/psychotherapy_cognitive_behavioural_therapy.htm) and the Royal College of Psychiatrists (www.rcpsych.ac.uk/mentalhealthinfoforall/treatments/cbt.aspx). Other useful websites are:

- www.babcp.com (British Association for Behavioural and Cognitive Psychotherapies)
- www.moodgym.anu.edu.au (information, quizzes, games and skills training to help prevent depression and low mood)
- www.livinglifetothefull.com (free online life skills courses)
- www.realhealth.org.uk (information about pain management and pain management courses to learn about CBT and how to implement it).

● complementary and alternative medicine

People who aren't helped by painkillers or don't like taking tablets sometimes turn to complementary and alternative medicine. Few of these treatments have been studied extensively in clinical trials, so it is difficult to assess whether complementary therapies are helpful for the pain caused by osteoarthritis and RA. If you are interested in trying complementary and alternative medicine therapies, discuss it with your doctor, nurse or physiotherapist. They will be able to help you decide what might be right for you, and save you a considerable amount of money if it's unlikely to help you.

Some common complementary and alternative treatments that have shown some promise for pain management in arthritis include:

- **Acupuncture:** This uses tiny needles which are inserted into your skin at precise points on the body. It is believed that the needles stimulate the body's energy channels and this helps to relieve pain. It is also believed that putting the needle into the skin stimulates the immune system to release chemicals in the body which help relieve pain. Studies of acupuncture for osteoarthritis of the knee have been mixed, but most have found some short-term relief of pain. Acupuncture is safe if you select a reputable practitioner, and use it whenever you have a flare-up as a way of managing your pain. Many physiotherapists are also trained to use acupuncture. All physio-therapists who practise acupuncture should be registered with the Acupuncture Association of Chartered Physiotherapists and can be found via their website, www.aacp.org.uk. Doctors who practise acupuncture will be registered with the British Medical Acu-puncture Society (www.medical-acupuncture.co.uk). Acupuncture is very safe, but may cause bruising and some discomfort where the needles are inserted into your skin.

- **Ginger:** Some research has found that ginger extract may be helpful in reducing pain in osteoarthritis, but it is unclear why this is so, and results have again been mixed. Side-effects of ginger supplements can include heartburn and diarrhoea. Talk to your doctor before taking ginger supplements, since they can interfere with prescription medications that thin your blood, such as warfarin.

- **Glucosamine and chondroitin:** Studies have been mixed on these nutritional supplements. Some have found benefits for people with osteoarthritis, but it has to be taken in high doses for a number of months. Don't use glucosamine if you are allergic to shellfish. Chondroitin sulphate may affect blood levels of warfarin if you are taking it.

- **Magnets:** Some people believe that placing magnets near your affected joint can relieve arthritic pain. Some small studies have found magnets can provide temporary pain relief, though others have found no benefit, and it isn't clear how magnet therapy works. A variety of magnetic products, such as bracelets, are available.

- **Tai chi and yoga:** These movement therapies involve gentle exercises and stretches combined with deep breathing. Many people use them to reduce stress, but some studies have found that tai chi and yoga may reduce pain in osteoarthritis. If you want to give tai chi or yoga a try, make sure you find a good instructor – ask for a recommendation from a friend or take a look at www.triyoga.co.uk. Avoid any moves that cause pain in your joints.

pain control and medication

If you are still in pain following good initial treatment of your OA, you may need to take some form of medication. If you have RA you will definitely need medication to suppress your inflammation. Don't assume that taking medication is all you need to do to get the most from your treatment. Continue exercising when possible and resting when you need to. If you are overweight, continue working to lose weight.

● *NSAIDs/COX-2 inhibitors*

- Non-steroidal anti-inflammatory drugs (NSAIDs) are the most commonly prescribed and widely used drugs for arthritis. They can relieve pain and reduce inflammation.

- Cox-2 inhibitors are a newer kind of NSAID that have fewer side effects on your stomach lining.

- NSAIDs work by blocking the activity of the enzyme cyclo-oxygenase, also known as COX. Research has shown that there are two forms, known as COX-1 and COX-2. NSAIDs affect both forms. COX-1 is involved in maintaining healthy tissue, while COX-2 is involved in the inflammation pathway.

- Over-the-counter NSAIDs include ibuprofen and naproxen sodium. Stronger versions of these NSAIDs and others are available by prescription.

- NSAIDs have risks of side-effects that increase when used at high dosages for long-term treatment. NICE recommends the inclusion of a PPI (proton pump inhibitor) to reduce the risk of side effects for people who are prescribed long term NSAIDs. These include gastric ulcers, cardiovascular problems, gastrointestinal bleeding, and liver and kidney damage. Consuming alcohol or taking steroids while using NSAIDs also increases your risk of gastrointestinal bleeding. Managing your medication and how and when you take it will limit these side-effects.

● *prescription painkillers*

If you have tried these treatments but are still experiencing severe pain and disability, you and your doctor can discuss other treatments. Stronger prescription analgesics (pain-relieving drugs) are available, including:

- Tramadol: this is an opioid and acts on the central nervous system to reduce your pain. It has no anti-inflammatory effects, but can provide effective pain relief with fewer side-effects than NSAIDs, though it may cause nausea, drowsiness and constipation. It is generally used for short-term treatment of acute flare-ups. Your doctor may recommend using it in combination with other drugs to increase pain relief.

- Prescription painkillers such as dihydracodeine, codeine and morphine: these may provide relief from more severe arthritic pain in both OA and RA.

These stronger medications can be addictive, but the risk is thought to be small in people who have severe pain. Side-effects may include nausea, constipation and drowsiness.

● *DMARDs*

The established drug management of rheumatoid arthritis is achieved through the use of disease-modifying drugs (DMARDs). They have also been labelled 'slow-acting anti-rheumatic drugs' (because they take weeks or months to work) and 'second-line agents'. Research has shown the effectiveness of early aggressive treatment with DMARDs in the treatment of RA. For some people, these drugs can stop disease progression and halt joint damage as well as manage their symptoms.

Examples of DMARDs include methotrexate, sulfasalazine, hydroxy-chloroquine (the anti-malarial), and Leflunomide. They can be used alone and are increasingly used in combination, which can be more effective than the use of one DMARD alone.

● biologics

These drugs are used to treat patients with RA who have not responded well to DMARDs. Anti-TNF is commonly used and works by blocking the inflammatory chemical in the body known as tumour necrosis factor alpha (TNF∝). A drug called Mabthera was approved by N.I.C.E in 2007 for people who didn't respond well to Anti-TNF. The biologic drugs currently available are either given by intravenous infusion or injected at home by the patient. Various new biologics have been licensed in the UK, but may or may not be available on the NHS for cost reasons, and others are under development – check the website of the National Rheumatoid Arthritis Society (www.rheumatoid.org.uk) for up-to-date information.

> **TIP**
>
> 'I hate taking medication and when I was diagnosed with RA at the age of 35, I found the thought of taking drugs for the rest of my life hard to deal with. When I realised the main reason was to prevent deformity of my joints, I found it the lesser evil.'   Sandra, RA, Scotland

● corticosteroid injections

Steroids are potent drugs which can reduce swelling and inflammation quickly. These drugs are closely related to cortisol, a hormone produced on the cortex of the adrenal glands. Injections of corticosteroid into your joint can be helpful in both osteoarthritis and RA. Doctors can prescribe short-term, high-dose intravenous steroids in some situations or locally into a specific joint for relief. You can also have intra-muscular injections of depomedrone for general pain relief.

Your doctor may limit the number of injections you can have each year, since too many steroid injections may cause joint damage.

● visco-supplementation

Visco-supplementation involves injections of hyaluronic acid into the knee and aims to provides a cushioning layer, in order to provide pain relief. This treatment is only approved for osteoarthritis of the knee, but its use in other joints is being researched. Injections are usually given weekly over several weeks and pain relief can last for a few months.

● surgery for osteoarthritis and RA

Surgery is generally reserved for severe osteoarthritis and RA that is not relieved by other treatments. You may consider surgery if your arthritis makes it very difficult to go about your daily tasks. Surgical treatments include:

- **Cleaning up the area around the joint (debridement):** Using arthroscopy, loose pieces of cartilage and bone are removed from around the joint to relieve pain. This is most useful if you have OA and are experiencing a locking sensation from a torn, roughened cartilage or loose debris in your knee joint.

- **Aspiration (fluid removal):** This is mainly used for swollen RA joints to remove the inflammatory fluid and help prevent joint damage.

- **Realigning bones (osteotomy):** Surgery to realign bones is typically used when joint replacement surgery isn't an option. Joint replacements are not usually done in younger people with OA as the new joints typically last 15–20 years and will then need replacing. If you have RA, joints will be replaced irrespective of age if there is a need. In an osteotomy, the surgeon cuts across the bone either above or below the joint to realign the limb. It is done most commonly to straighten the knee and can reduce pain by transferring the force of the joint away from the worn-out part of the knee.

- **Fusing bones (arthrodesis):** Surgeons can also permanently fuse bones in a joint to increase stability and reduce pain. The fused joint, such as an ankle, can then bear weight with improved stability and reduced pain. The joint has no flexibility and if you have severe joint damage from RA your pain may still persist.

- **Joint replacement (arthroplasty):** Joint replacement surgery can help you to resume an active, pain-free lifestyle if you have OA. The surgeon removes the damaged joint surfaces and replaces them with plastic and metal surfaces called prostheses. In RA joint replacement can help reduce your pain, but functional activity improvements will always depend on the level of control of the inflammation. The hip and knee joints (see figs 2.5 and 2.6) are the most commonly replaced joints, but you can also have your shoulder, elbow, finger or ankle joints replaced. In smaller hand joints, joint replacement can improve appearance if you have RA, and may also improve your joint mobility. How long your new joint will last depends on how you use it: artificial joints can wear or come loose, and eventually may need to be replaced. Some knee and hip joints can last 20 years. The surgery carries a small risk of infection and bleeding.

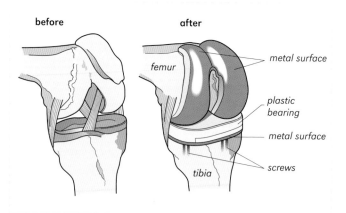

Figure 2.5 Knee joint replacement

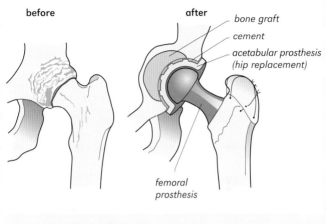

before

after
- bone graft
- cement
- acetabular prosthesis (hip replacement)

femoral prosthesis

Figure 2.6 Hip joint replacement

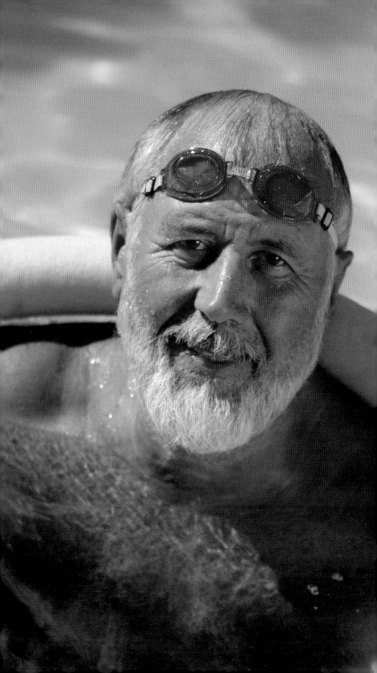

part 3
the exercises

where do I start?
Whether you have osteoarthritis or RA, regular gentle exercise can improve the range of movement in a joint and ease stiffness. Movement puts changing pressures through the cartilage and the joint, which helps the circulation and the synovial fluid to 'oil' the joint. In RA this may not be true if the cartilage is severely damaged or eroded.

Everyone has heard the 'no pain no gain theory', but this will do little to encourage you to exercise and step onto the path to personal fitness. Some people do nothing, or fear that exercise will make them feel worse; others do too much and feel terrible. Your personality and experience of exercise will influence how you react. Exercise doesn't have to hurt, and physical pain can be avoided if you exercise within your ability. However, it can be hard at first to change your habits and become disciplined with a commitment to exercise! You should expect muscular aches after exercise, but pain can and should be avoided.

the benefits of exercise

Regular exercise can not only help your arthritis but help you to:

- reduce the risk of dying prematurely from heart disease
- reduce the risk of developing diabetes
- reduce the risk of developing high blood pressure
- reduce blood pressure in people who already have it
- reduce feelings of depression and anxiety
- control weight
- build and maintain healthy bones, muscles, and joints
- in the elderly, improve strength and balance which reduces the risk of falling.

For the greatest overall benefits, it is recommended that you do 20 to 30 minutes of aerobic activity three or more times a week, and some type of muscle strengthening activity, as well as stretching, twice a week. If you can't manage this, you can still see great improvements by trying to include two or three 10-minute sessions, adding up to 30 minutes of moderate intensity every day. This can include walking, hoovering, climbing the stairs, pushing a shopping trolley or even cleaning! It is important to remember this when you are having a flare-up and your exercise tolerance is affected by pain. Little and often will still make a difference.

The first part of this section is intended to help those new to exercise, and those with some 'no' answers in their MOT. I have treated many people with both OA and RA at my clinic and they have enjoyed steady progress when following this routine to get them started and improve their general level of fitness. I have included three programmes here: a home workout programme (page 67) that you can use to get started, a water-based programme (page 80), which is helpful when your joints are sore, and a walking programme. This is followed by a series of specific exercises for improving the strength of your joints. Don't worry if you haven't exercised much in the past. What is important are the different needs you will have depending on experience, the inflammatory phases of your arthritis and levels of pain.

If you have never exercised before, you should start with the 'Steady beginnings' programme on pages 69–76, which will start you off gently on improving your overall fitness so you don't do too much too soon and risk a flare-up. If you have exercised before but are coming back after time out or an inflammatory episode you will also benefit from reading this section. Even as an experienced sufferer of arthritis, you will benefit from a change to your usual routine.

anytime, anywhere exercises

It is important to be able to fit exercise into your routine, whether you are watching TV, or sitting at work or in the car. Here are some ideas for exercises you can try to fit into your daily routine however busy you are.

- Balance on one leg when you are cleaning your teeth, waiting in a queue or waiting at the photocopier.
- Kick your shoes off at work and do your foot intrinsic exercises (page 112).
- Lift your pelvic floor whenever you are sitting at traffic lights or going upstairs.
- Do 10 squats (page 70) every time you go to the toilet.
- Do 10 knee extensions (page 108) every time you sit down.
- Do 10 clams before you get out of bed every morning. You can use the duvet as a weight!
- Do your heel raises (page 113) as you wash up.
- Squeeze socks in your hands (page 100) while watching TV.

before you start

set your exercise goals

Now that you have decided to exercise in order to help manage your arthritis, it's helpful to set yourself a goal and work out what will ensure you achieve it. A goal will help keep you motivated and think twice about skipping an exercise session! Be realistic about the goals that you set for yourself. Don't aim too high and risk the disappointment of failure, or so low that the exercise has little effect and presents no challenge or personal achievement. This section includes a wide range of exercises and stretches to keep you on track. You may prefer to join an exercise class, which is a great way to keep you motivated.

It is important not to overestimate your current level of fitness. Be honest with yourself and you will make sure that you start at the right pace for you and progress quickly without any setbacks due to flare-up, pain or illness. If you are an experienced exerciser looking to increase the amount of training you are doing, it is just as important to be as realistic as a complete beginner. Doing too much too soon will cause you pain so it is important not to overdo it. Even when you are feeling fit, be careful not to do too much, and pace yourself (see page 36). Problems and flare-ups can arise at any time and may become an issue if you don't monitor both your exercise plan and your day-to-day life. Stress, deadlines at work, moving house, even gardening over a sunny weekend are all things that can impact on activity levels without you realising, until you experience a flare-up and realise you have pushed your body too far.

medication and medical conditions

If you have any other diagnosed medical conditions it doesn't mean you can't exercise. However, check with your doctor that you will not do yourself any harm. Most medical conditions will benefit from exercise – you may just need to be monitored until your level of fitness improves. If you are taking medication that affects your metabolism (for example for diabetes and thyroid problems) you may need to monitor the effect of exercise until you get used to training. Again, if you have any concerns chat to your doctor.

If you think you may have any biomechanical anomalies such as flat feet, scoliosis (curvature of the spine), uncontrolled pain or a leg length discrepancy, you should see a physiotherapist or a podiatrist for an assessment before you start exercising, as insoles and other appliances are available which can make things much easier for you.

pregnancy and post-natal exercise

If you are currently pregnant, you can still exercise and carry on as long as you feel well enough to do so. As you get bigger you may find it less comfortable, but you can still exercise.

If you have RA and have had to stop taking your medication during your pregnancy, you should exercise, but with caution. Many women find pregnancy helps their symptoms, but it is important not to overdo things.

If you have just had a baby, it is important that you have had your post-natal checks and have restarted your disease-modifying drugs before starting to exercise again. You need to make sure your tummy muscles are recovering and that you are doing your pelvic floor exercises. A good bra is even more important at this time. If you are breastfeeding your size will fluctuate, which makes getting a well-fitting bra difficult. Get measured for a sports bra in a good department store or specialist bra shop, and try to get measured when your breasts are at their fullest. A second 'pull over' soft bra or sports top with a built in bra/crop top will provide more support, and allow for any fluctuation in size. For further advice on bras visit www.lessbounce.co.uk or www.bravissimo.co.uk.

current flare-ups and infections

If you are suffering from a flare-up, pain, cough or cold, wait until you feel better before you start a new exercise programme. After a cold it is important to return to exercise slowly, as your immune system will still be recovering. Take it easy, as the last thing you need is another cold! With RA your immune system is already compromised so it doesn't need any unnecessary stress.

exercise and arthritis – key points
Exercise can help reduce the symptoms of arthritis, but an inflamed, hot or painful RA joint needs rest.

- Exercise programmes should be devised in consultation with your doctor, physiotherapist or health or fitness professional.
- Don't exercise a painful, inflamed or hot joint. You can move the joint gently through its range of movement several times to help reduce stiffness and improve circulation.
- Start gently and increase the intensity of your exercise programme gradually over weeks or months.
- Warm up thoroughly beforehand. Cool down after exercise with gentle stretches.
- Pay attention to good technique and try to move smoothly. Don't force a joint – your range will increase the more you practise.
- If your joint feels particularly painful afterwards, take it more slowly at your next exercise session.
- If an activity causes you pain or increases your pain beyond what is normal, stop straight away.
- Try whenever you can to add activity into your life – walk to nearby shops instead of driving, and take the stairs instead of using the lift or escalator.

checking your progress
Nothing will motivate you to keep exercising more than seeing how you have improved without even noticing! These quick and simple tests that you can perform on yourself, or with a little help, will allow you to map your progress every four to six weeks. Prepare to be amazed by how much you can improve in the first six weeks.

range of movement self-tests
These are simple but effective ways for you to monitor your joints' range of movement. Make a note of the measurements and the date,

and four to six weeks after you have started your exercise programme take the measurements again. It's a great motivator to see what exercise can do for your joints.

1 Shoulder movement

Hold a ruler in your hand. Stand with your back against a wall and lift your arm out in front of you and then, if you can, over your head. Once the ruler touches the wall, slide your hand down the ruler towards the wall and measure the point you reach. Next time measure to see if you can get closer. If you have stiff or sore shoulders and know you can't lift them over your head, use a pen instead. Lift your arm as high as you can and make a mark on the wall. To track your progress you can put a sheet of paper on the inside of a wardrobe and date each mark.

2 Hip movement

Lie on a double bed and gently move both your legs away from each other. If you can get one heel to the edge of the bed you only need to take one measurement, and that is where the other leg reaches. You may need help to take this measurement with a tape measure, but simply measure the distance between both your ankles.

3 Knee joints

Sit on your bed with your legs supported and stretched out in front of you. Bend both your knees, keep your feet on the bed and move your heels towards your bottom. When you can't bend them any further, measure the distance between your heel and your bottom.

4 Forward bending

This will measure how much forward bending movement you have in your back and hips. Simply slide your hands slowly down the front of your legs. Stop when you reach your limit – never push too far or bounce. You may have a convenient freckle on your leg to remind you how far you can reach; if not, use a ruler to measure how far away your fingertips are from the floor.

5 Hands

This is a good way to keep a check on your hands and the small joints in your fingers. Place a ruler in the palm of your hand and bend your fingers to make a fist, or touch the palm of your hand. If you can't touch your palm, measure how far your fingers are from touching.

6 Finger and thumb joints

This is another test of the flexibility in your finger and thumb joints. Aim to touch the pads of each finger to the pad of your thumb. If you can't, measure how far apart your thumb and finger are in each case.

fitness self-tests

All of these tests are simple and easy to do. Set a clock to time one minute and do as many repetitions as you can, but don't attempt to time yourself until you are happy that you can do the exercises safely. If you need to rest, do so, especially if you have RA, and remember to pace yourself. Make a note of how many repetitions you have managed each time you do the tests, as a way of monitoring your progress over the coming weeks when you add exercise into your life.

step-ups

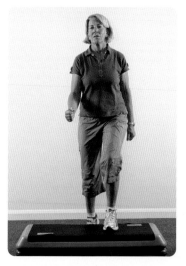

- Use any step. If you don't have stairs at home you could use the kerb at the side of the road.
- Use the banister or wall for balance if you need to.
- Step up with your right foot first, ensuring your whole foot is on the step, then bring your left foot up alongside it.
- Step down with your right leg, bringing the left foot to join it.
- Repeat, leading with your left leg.

press-ups (against a wall, bench, window ledge or kitchen worktop)

- Place your hands shoulder width apart on the surface of your choice.
- Step your feet away from the surface and rest your weight through your hands.
- Slowly bend your elbows and lower your chest towards the wall or surface.
- Push yourself away from the wall or surface.
- Make sure you don't arch your back.

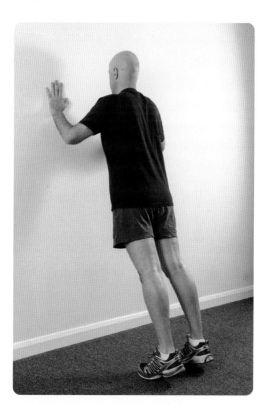

squats

- Stand with your feet hip distance apart, and reach your arms out in front of you to help you balance.
- Bend your knees as far as you comfortably can, as if you are going to sit down.
- Keep your knees behind your toes and stick your bottom out behind you.

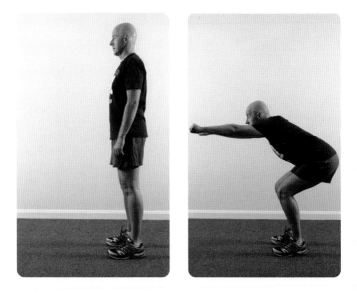

If you prefer, you can use walking as a way of seeing how much you have improved. Time yourself walking a set distance (count the number of times you need to rest). Soon you will be able to walk the distance without a rest.

Alternatively you can pick any exercise from pages 69–76 of this book and count the number of repetitions you can do in one minute. Remember you can rest as many times as you need to. The rest breaks will reduce as your fitness improves.

steady beginnings: home routine

You may be surprised by how much exercise you can do at home. You don't need to build an extension for your own gym or to buy expensive equipment. Investing in small weights of 1–5kg, resistance bands and putty is a great place to start. You can use putty, which is available in different strengths, to strengthen the muscles in your hands. All these take up minimal space.

If you do have space, you can invest in an exercise bike or cross-trainer to use at home. This will encourage you to exercise even when the weather is bad or allow you to fit exercise into your day when it suits you. Many people like to spend 10 minutes on the exercise bike before getting dressed in the morning. There are many models of home exercise equipment that can be folded away.

> **TIP**
>
> 'I had used exercise putty with my physio at the hospital, but I find making bread is just as good for exercising my hands. I can't do it everyday but once a week is good enough and great to do with my grandchildren.'
>
> Margaret, OA, London

Getting the right pair of trainers is one of the most important things you can do when you start to exercise. Make sure you take the time to find out what your 'foot type' is – a good trainer shop can help you with this. Some people have flat feet and need more of an arch support in their trainers. If your feet are badly affected by arthritis you may need a special insole made by a podiatrist. A cushioned insole may help to make the small joints of your feet feel more comfortable. Many of my patients use off-the-shelf insoles or gel inserts, which are available from most high street chemists.

You can buy exercise equipment from most sports shops or from Argos or department stores. You can also order equipment and gel insoles from www.physiosupplies.co.uk.

to gym or not to gym?

You don't need an expensive gym membership and lots of time to get fit. Many of us are too broke, or too busy to go to the gym. Gyms can seem intimidating and unfriendly places where the 'in-crowd' get all the help and attention while those who are really in need of help are ignored. If this is how you feel, take control and exercise when and where it suits you and your lifestyle. It's not important where you exercise; just make sure you do it!

This set of exercise ideas is designed to help you return to fitness, whether you are a beginner or returning to exercise after a flare-up, and will complement the specific strengthening and range of movement exercises later in this book. The simple routine – I don't like to call it a programme as it is not intended to be that regimented – will build up noticeable pace and stamina in only a few weeks. Try doing the full routine (steps 1–9) three times a week, and you will be impressed with your results. Once this becomes easy, progress to the walking or swimming programmes (pages 77 and 80) and see your fitness improve even more.

preparing to exercise at home

Exercising at home needs minimal preparation – put aside some time every day, or grab a spare five minutes when you can.

- Choose a time of day which suits you.
- Try to eat around two hours before exercising – too soon after eating can make you feel nauseous.
- Clear a space – move the coffee table or anything you could trip over out of the way.
- Wear comfortable clothes and supportive shoes – trainers are best.
- Make sure the room isn't too hot – open a window.

- Have some water to hand in case you get thirsty.
- Make sure you won't be interrupted, and turn off your mobile phone!
- Stick some motivating music on, and get moving.

warm-up and stretching

march on the spot

1 March on the spot to warm up. Start at a moderate pace that you can maintain for the time suggested. Swing your arms and lift your knees high. You should aim to become breathless, but still be able to talk easily.

- week 1: march for 2 minutes
- week 2: march for 4 minutes
- week 3: march for 6 minutes

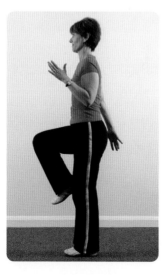

squats

2 Stand with your feet hip distance apart and your hands on your hips. Squat as if to sit down, and then stand tall, hands on your hips or out in front of you.

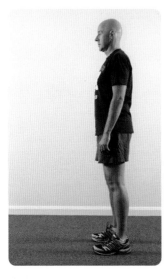 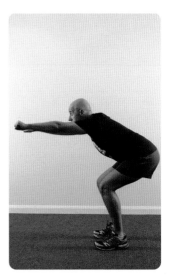

- week 1: sit to stand 5 times
- week 2: sit to stand 10 times
- week 3: sit to stand 15 times

step back lunge

3 Stand with your feet hip distance apart and your hands on your hips. Step back with one leg, as far as you would if you were walking backwards, then return it to the starting position. Repeat 5–15 times, holding the final step back and keeping your heel on the floor. Hold for 30 seconds, then repeat with the other leg. You will feel the stretch in the back of your leg.

- week 1: step back 5 times
- week 2: step back 10 times
- week 3: step back 15 times

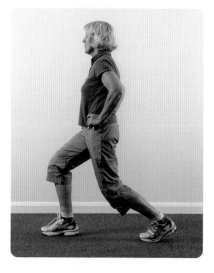

aerobic exercises

As you improve you can add aerobic exercise, which will increase your heart rate and fat burning. All these exercises can be mixed and matched to make up a personal routine. If one exercise causes you pain, substitute another one.

step-ups

4   Step-ups can be performed on a small box or at the bottom of your staircase. Step up and down with one leg 5–15 times and then change legs. This is one 'set' or repetition. Continue for 2–6 sets with one minute's rest between each set. Maintain good posture by standing up tall with your shoulders back, looking straight ahead, and keep sipping water between sets so you do not dehydrate.

- week 1: step up 5 times for 2 sets
- week 2: step up 10 times for 4 sets
- week 3: step up 15 times for 6 sets

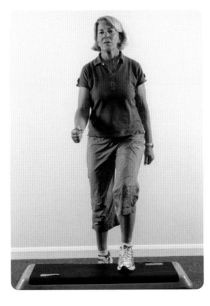

bicep curl and press

5 Strengthening your arms with bicep curls and an overhead press will help improve your overall strength and posture. Hold a weight in each hand (see box), starting with 0.5–2 kg weights depending on your level of fitness. Stand tall and alternate your arms, bending your arm from your side to your shoulder then pushing the weight above your head. Repeat 5–15 times for one set. Continue for 2 to 4 sets with a minute's rest between sets.

- week 1: lift 5 times for 2 sets
- week 2: lift 10 times for 3 sets
- week 3: lift 15 times for 4 sets

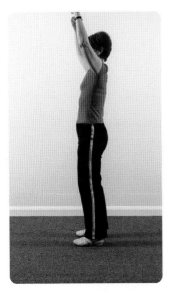
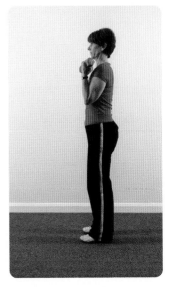
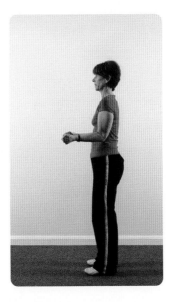

weights

You don't have to buy expensive weights: you can use tins of beans (400 g) or bags of sugar (1 kg) as weights in each hand. If you want to buy weights, start with light weights and progress as you become stronger. You can buy beginner's sets of 1–5 kg weights from most sports stores, but don't try to lift too much too soon.

side bends

6 Holding your home-made weights in each hand, keep your arms by your sides. Slowly lean over to the right, allowing your hand to reach your mid-thigh. Bring the other arm up and over your head. Repeat 5–15 times and then repeat on the left side. This is one set. After one minute's rest continue for up to 6 sets.

- week 1: bend to each side 5 times for 2 sets
- week 2: bend to each side 10 times for 4 sets
- week 3: bend to each side 15 times for 6 sets

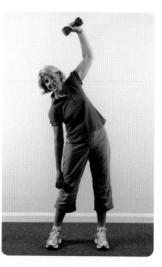

winding down and toning stretches

march on the spot

7 March on the spot slowly, concentrating on your posture and lifting your knees. Breathe deeply in and out. This will allow your heart rate to return to normal as you keep moving and allow your body to cool down gradually.

- week 1: march for 2 minutes
- week 2: march for 4 minutes
- week 3: march for 6 minutes

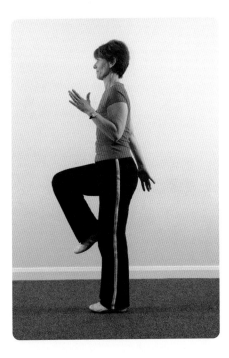

hip stretch

8 Stand with your hands resting on a kitchen surface or the back of a steady chair. Lift one leg out behind you, making sure you don't arch your back, and lift the foot off the floor. Squeeze your bottom as you lift. Repeat 5–15 times and then change legs.

- week 1: lift each leg back 5 times
- week 2: lift each leg back 10 times
- week 3: lift each leg back 15 times

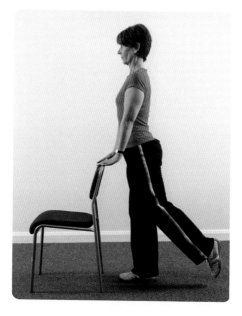

9 Stand up straight, and take six deep breaths in through your nose. Breathe out through your mouth, making sure you empty your lungs, and gently lift your pelvic floor. You will feel your lower tummy gently tighten as you do this, working your core muscles which protect the spine.

TIP

'I used to hate the thought of exercising when I was in pain, but when I learnt how to pace myself I realised just how much stronger my joints could be. It doesn't make the flare-ups any less painful, but I recover from them much easier now.'

Frank, RA, Yorkshire

steady beginnings: walking

Walking is not a soft option. You can actually burn more calories walking than running, if you vary your walking speed and style. It is a particularly good way to ease into exercise if you are unfit, or recovering from a flare-up, as it is a low impact exercise; it also gets you out in the fresh air, and it's free!

Initially, follow the 'little and often' rule and you will see the results add up. You can walk more by getting off the bus or train one stop early, or buy your lunch from a shop further away from work. Try using a pedometer, so you can monitor how many steps you take each day, and see if you can gradually increase the number.

Alternatively, if you have severe RA or are in pain you may prefer to start your walking programme on a treadmill or a cross-trainer at the gym. Both of these allow you to exercise with less impact, and also mean that you will not be stranded out and about and far from home should you feel the need to stop. This allows the body to adapt gradually to the stresses of exercise and helps you to avoid injury.

When walking, try to maintain a good posture from head to toe, with your head up and shoulders back, keeping your steps steady so you can keep up an even pace. Swinging your arms helps speed up your pace, and to progress as you get fitter you can swing your arms while holding weights. Make sure you wear supportive footwear or trainers. Any running shop can give you advice on the right trainer for your foot type, which considers the shape and width of your foot and the height of your arch.

walk safe

It is important to choose walking routes that are safe. If you plan to walk on your own, walk when it is light and when places are busy and not in secluded areas. Get into the habit of leaving a note at home with the time you left for your walk, where you are going and when you are due home. Take your mobile phone with you so you are always in contact.

walking programme

This simple routine will build up visible pace and stamina in only a few weeks.

weeks 1–2

Start by walking every day. This may be as simple as walking to the station, getting off the bus one stop early or walking to buy your lunch. Taking the stairs instead of the lift also counts as walking and may be possible more than once a day.

weeks 3–4

You have already added walking into your routine without taking up any extra time in weeks 1 and 2. Now think about adding an extra 15 minute walk into each day. This may be part of your route to work, to the shops or to a friend's home for coffee. You could offer to walk a neighbour's dog or give a new mother a break by taking her baby for a walk.

weeks 5–6

Increase your daily walking time to 20 minutes in week 5 and 30 minutes in week 6. You can use this time to switch off and have time to yourself, or if you prefer make phone calls and catch up with all those friends you never get round to calling back. Better still, get a friend to walk with you and spend quality time while walking.

weeks 7–8

Now you have an established routine of daily walking, it is time to speed things up a little. Introduce swinging your arms and focus on striding out as you walk. See how much further you can walk once you increase your pace. A pedometer will help you monitor your distance. Alternatively you could simply use a route you have walked previously in 30 minutes and aim to walk beyond the original finish point.

weeks 9–10

Now you should be noticing changes in your fitness and your waistline. You are ready to progress, and introducing uphill and downhill walking is a great way to improve your cardiovascular fitness. Find a hill either in a park or a street, and walk up without stopping. Use the walk back down to get your breath back. You will still be working your muscles, just in a different way. You can make this a 15 minute part of your work-out – walking to and from the hill is a good warm-up and cool-down.

weeks 11–12

Another way to progress is to walk while holding weights. These don't have to cost money and can be two tins of beans! Walk your regular routes and focus on your pace and arm swing. To make sure your grip remains strong, secure the weights to your hands with loops of elastic. Slip the loop of elastic over your hand and place the can of beans under the elastic in your palm. To have a mixed workout over the week, vary your programme each day – one day with weights, one day with hills and one day on the flat.

exercising in water

Warm water exercise (hydrotherapy) is particularly helpful when you have RA as the warmth can help ease your joint pain and make movement easier. Exercise of any kind in water is great because your body weight is supported and the resistance of moving through the water improves muscle strength and endurance. Stretching, walking and moving floats through water exercises your joints without putting them under strain.

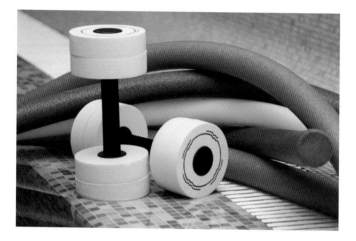

the benefits

Research has shown that exercising in water can improve your health and fitness. Exercising for just 12 weeks is all it takes to start seeing results such as:

- increased muscle strength

- improved mood and quality of sleep

- reduced fear of exercise

- greater flexibility

- loss of excess body fat

- reduced risk of exercise-related injuries.

There are a range of exercise in water classes to choose from, including:

- **Hydrotherapy** – a type of exercise therapy offered by physio-therapists. The water for hydrotherapy sessions is usually heated to around 34°C. Group sessions or one-on-one training are available – check with your physiotherapist or ask your GP to refer you. At these sessions you will be in chest-deep water, which allows your arms and legs to float and move with the help of the water. This is especially beneficial if your muscles are weak or you are in a lot of pain. As you become stronger you can exercise with floats that will offer resistance to your movement through the water.

- **Gentle water exercise** – many sports centres and pools offer gentle water exercise programmes for people who are elderly, disabled or unfit.

- **Gentle aqua aerobics** – many sports centres and pools offer exercise classes in water that aim to improve general fitness. Because aqua aerobics exercises can be a bit more vigorous than hydrotherapy, the water is cooler.

Contact your local hospital physiotherapy department and ask if they offer hydrotherapy or other water exercise sessions. You may need to get your GP to refer you for treatment, but there are some private hydro-therapy pools that you can visit and pay per session. If you have RA your specialist can refer you.

Before you join a class:

- Always check with your doctor or physiotherapist before you start. You may need to avoid certain movements if you have had joint replacement surgery recently or in the past. Think carefully about the venue. Public swimming pools, for example, generally have cooler water, so you could feel cold while exercising.

- Is the pool easy to access? Is there a hoist? Are the changing rooms accessible and comfortable?

- Before choosing a class, make sure it is appropriate to your level of fitness and ability. Go and watch a class before you attend.

safety when exercising in warm water

The combination of exercise and warm water can make you tired, so keep this in mind when you are planning your day.

- It will take time to build up your fitness, so exercise for no more than 15 minutes at first. Increase to 30 minutes as your fitness improves.

- If you are exercising in a hot spa, get out after 5 minutes or so.

- If you feel light-headed, sick or dizzy at any stage, get out of the water.

- Don't try to do too much too soon. If you feel out of breath, slow down.

- Perform each movement as smoothly as you can.

- Ask your physiotherapist to prescribe you an individual hydro-therapy programme.

- Keep the body part you are exercising under the water. This may mean you need to squat at times.

- If a movement causes pain stop, slow down, and be more gentle.

- If the pool has water jets you can use these to massage your joints and muscles.

- Drink plenty of fluids while you are exercising in the water and afterwards.

- Rest for a while when you get home.

- If you have painful joints or sore muscles for more than a few hours after your class, do less and take it more slowly next time.

---

safety point

● Check with your doctor if you have particular medical problems – such as heart disease, low blood pressure or diabetes – before you do any exercises in warm water.

---

hydrotherapy programme

These are exercises that you can do in your local swimming or hydrotherapy pool. Contact your local hospital physiotherapy department and ask if they offer hydrotherapy sessions and how they are organised: most do, and a referral from your GP is all you need. There are some private hydrotherapy pools, but this depends on where you live. How the sessions are arranged will vary from area to area – some will be supervised and some will allow you to do your own thing.

shoulder exercise: give yourself a hug

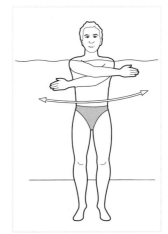

1 Stand in water at chest height with your arms stretched out in front of you on the surface of the water.

2 Keeping your arms straight, open them wide out to each side, then back to the centre, crossing them in front of you.

3 As you repeat this opening and closing of your arms, move your hands deeper into the water towards your hips. This makes the exercise harder as it adds resistance from the water. Holding floats or paddles will increase the resistance even further.

Repeat 10 times.

elbow exercise: water boxing

1 Stand in water deep enough to cover your shoulders and allow your arms to sit on the surface of the water.

2 Reach one arm forwards in front of you as you bend the other behind you.

3 You can put floats under your forearms to help with buoyancy.

Repeat 10 times.

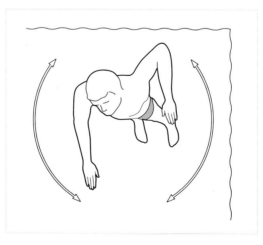

back exercise: do the twist

1 Stand holding onto the handrail in chest-deep water.

2 Bring your knees together against the wall with your knees bent at right angles.

3 Swing both feet up to the right elbow and then over to the left elbow.

Repeat 10–15 times.

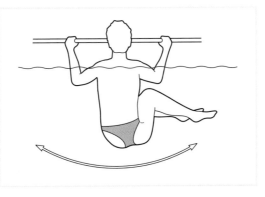

back exercise: the pendulum

1 Lie on your back holding onto the handrail and allow your body to float.

2 Bending at the waist, and keep your legs together, sweep both your legs from side to side on the surface of the water.

3 You can use a float under your thighs to help with buoyancy.

Repeat 10 times.

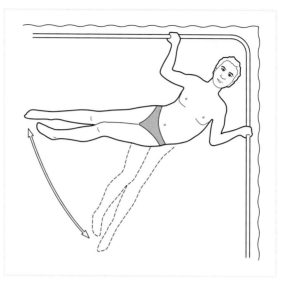

hip exercise: march on the spot

1 Stand in chest-deep water. Bend alternating knees towards your chest.

2 Clap your hands under your thigh as you lift each leg.

Repeat 10–15 times.

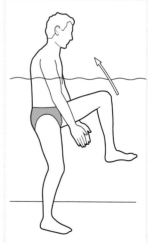

knee exercise: kick your butt

1 Stand up straight in chest-deep water and hold the handrail.

2 Bend your knee, bringing your foot towards your bottom as high as you can.

3 Lower your foot back to the floor.

Repeat 10–15 times for each leg.

You can make this harder by adding a float around your ankle.

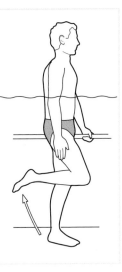

ankle exercise: heel raises

1 Stand with your shoulders under the water.

2 If you need help with your balance, hold onto the side of the pool.

3 Push yourself up onto your toes, lifting your heels off the floor then lowering them back down again.

Repeat 10 times.

You can progress this by walking up and down the pool on your tiptoes.

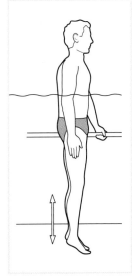

strengthening exercises

This part of the book includes specific exercises to strengthen your muscles and keep your joints supple. This will help you manage and reduce your joint pain. You may have done some of them before and some may be new to you. If you are nervous about exercising while in pain, take it slowly – you will not do yourself any harm or make your pain worse.

choosing your exercises

Here are some suggestions for different times when your arthritis may be more painful than others.

When you are in severe pain:

- consider the hydrotherapy exercises or the swimming programme – this will help keep you moving but is gentle, and if you pace yourself will not make your pain worse
- pole dancing, especially lying down (page 106)
- transverse abdominis (page 103)
- bicep curls without weights (page 97)
- knee extensions without weights (page 108)
- finger exercises in warm/cold water (page 101)
- feet intrinsics (page 112).

As things start to improve:

- pace yourself through the walking or swimming programmes as you feel able – though stay with week 1 for another week or two if that suits you
- spine stretch (page 93)
- pole dancing, standing or sitting (page 106)
- chin tucks (page 91)
- start on the flare-up and beginner's routine (page 69).

Aim to exercise for 15 minutes every day if you feel able to.

As you are ready to progress:

- get moving with either the walking or swimming programme – alternate different weeks if you like variety – or start on the running programme if you are ready for that
- knee extensions with weights (page 108)
- cat stretch (page 105)
- overhead press (page 96)
- resistance band exercises (page 98).

At this stage you can try any of the other exercises in this book, and aim to exercise for 15–30 minutes daily. You can do different exercises every day if you like, but by now you will probably have your favourites!

neck and upper back

Keeping a full and active range of movement in the neck and back is important for function and pain control. These simple exercises will help to gently stretch the muscles around the upper spine and neck and allow you to maintain a full range of movement.

hold–relax stretch

1 Gently push the side of your head into your hand and hold for 10 seconds.

2 Relax from pushing into your hand and gently stretch your neck, moving your ear towards your shoulder. Hold this stretch for 5 seconds and repeat on the other side.

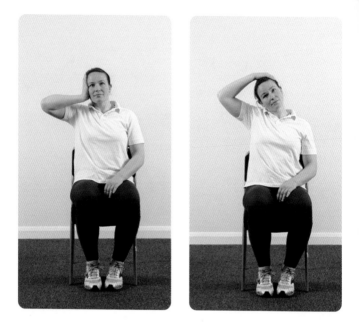

Variation: This same stretch can be used to help rotation in your neck:

1 Gently push your cheek into your hand as you try and turn your head.

2 Hold for 10 seconds, relax and then turn your head further to the right or left.

3 Repeat this hold and relax process until you feel you have reached your comfortable limit of movement.

chin tucks

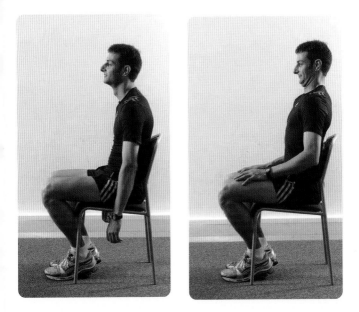

This is a great exercise to improve your posture and reduce stiffness at the base of your neck and the top of your spine. You can do this sitting down at work or lying in bed. Take care with this exercise if you have RA and any instability in your neck or have had recent neck surgery.

1 Make sure you have a good sitting or lying posture.

2 Drop your chin slightly to give yourself a double chin and keep your head in this position.

3 Gently push the tip of your tongue into the roof of your mouth.

4 If you are sitting, move your head backwards; if you are lying down, push your head into the supporting surface.

5 Hold this position for 2–3 seconds then relax your tongue and your chin.

6 Never push into pain and keep it slow and gentle at all times.

Variation: The harder option is to work with resistance:

1 Lie on your back with your head on a firm pillow or gym ball.

2 Push your head into the pillow or the ball, and relax.

3 Slowly turn your head from side to side as you maintain your double chin.

---

what is a gym ball?
This is a large inflatable ball that you can use to help you stretch and exercise, and it also makes a great chair to encourage good posture. The taller you are, the bigger the ball you will need. You can buy them from Argos, most large department stores and also online. Expect to pay about £25 at most.

spine stretch

Lying on a rolled towel for 15–20 minutes every night before you go to sleep is a great stretch for your spine between the shoulder blades, and also your chest muscles. If this area is stiff or tight it will affect the movement in your shoulders.

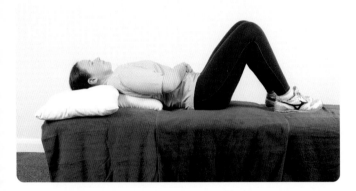

1 Roll up a towel so it has a diameter of 10–15 cm and secure it with rubber bands.

2 Lie on your back on a bed with the towel lengthways down your spine, from the base of your neck to the middle of your back.

3 Raise your arms to either side of your head and let them rest on the bed. If this is too much of a stretch, rest your arms on pillows to reduce the pull across your chest.

Variation: You can achieve the same stretch by lying over a gym ball.

shoulders, elbows, wrists and hands

pulley over the door frame

Arthritis commonly affects the shoulder joints, and a combination of pain and stiffness makes movement difficult. Using a pulley helps movement and stretching of the shoulders. You can buy pulleys from medical suppliers (see page 118) or make one from a dressing gown cord.

1 Sit on a chair with a hook overhead to hang the pulley from.

2 Pulling down with your left hand will help movement of the right shoulder.

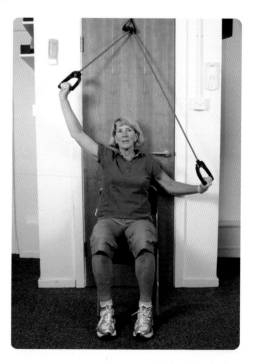

shoulder shrugs

This is a gentle exercise to help the shoulders and neck, and is safe to use even during a flare-up. You can make it easier or harder by adding weights of between 2 and 5 kg.

1 Standing or sitting, pull your shoulders up towards your ears.

2 Keep your elbows straight throughout, especially if you are holding weights.

3 Hold this position for 5 seconds, then slowly lower your shoulders.

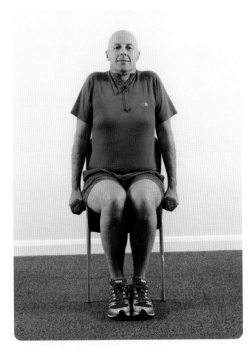

Variation: When your arthritis is less painful you can use weights to increase your muscle strength. If you have a weak grip, you can use resistance bands to hold the weights in place, or you can buy weights that have straps attached to help you grip them.

Repeat 10 times for one set and do 2 sets.

overhead press

You can do this sitting or standing. Either way, make sure you have your weight evenly spread between both feet or buttocks.

1 Holding the weights of your choice in your hands, place your hands at shoulder height.

2 Slowly raise your hands over your head, then lower your hands back to your shoulders.

Repeat 5–10 times for one set, and do 3 sets.

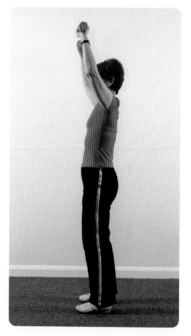

bicep curls

You can do this exercise sitting or standing. It's a great way to strengthen your arms and hands while keeping your elbows flexible.

1 Hold a can of soup or beans in each hand.

2 Slowly bend and straighten your elbows, taking your hands to your shoulders and then back down to your sides.

Variations: You can use no weights when your joints are sore or inflamed, or as you get stronger you can use bags of sugar or invest in small dumbbells.

Repeat 5 times on each arm for one set, and repeat this set 3 times. Alternatively, each time you do this exercise you can note down how many you can do, and try to equal or beat this number next time.

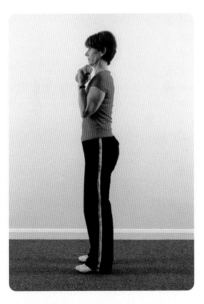

press-ups

Press-ups are great for strengthening the muscles around the shoulders and upper back. You can easily adjust this exercise to your level of fitness as you become stronger: start by pressing away from a wall, and progress through to using the kitchen worktop or a park bench, to the floor.

See page 65 for instructions and photos.

resistance band pull-ups

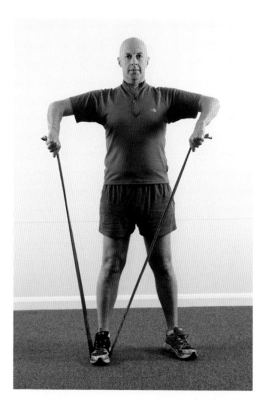

This is a great exercise for your hands, wrists, elbows and shoulders. Resistance bands take up very little space and can fit into your bag or pocket, enabling you to use them to exercise outside. To make them more comfortable to hold, use the hand grips that you can buy with them, or make your own from foam lagging for pipes, which you can buy from any hardware shop.

1 Hold each end of a resistance band and loop the band under your feet.

2 Pull up on the band so your hands are level with your chin. Keep your knees straight and your weight equal between both feet.

3 Slowly allow your arms to return to your sides.

Repeat 10 times for one set and do 3 sets.

Variation: You can make this harder by using a stronger resistance band or making the one you have shorter.

praying stretch

This is a great exercise to increase the range of movement in your wrists and stretch the muscles in your forearms.

1 Sit with your elbows on a table and your palms together.

2 Hold the stretch for five seconds, then slowly slide your elbows apart.

Repeat five times.

socks in hands

This is a great exercise to do while watching TV. You can use socks or a sponge ball, but if you are going through a flare-up and your hands are painful, you can use a gel ice pack to help with pain and inflammation. It's a great way to stretch and strengthen the muscles in your hands.

1 Roll up a pair of socks so they fit into the palm of your hand.

2 Slowly squeeze your fingers into the socks and towards your palm.

3 Make sure you squeeze your thumb into the socks too, as the muscles of the thumb are important for gripping strength.

finger stretches

After a flare-up, the small joints in the fingers and hands can be stiff and sore. This is a great way to get them moving and improve functional strength in your hands. You can make it easier or more difficult by varying the size and resistance of the elastic band. Alternatively you can squeeze putty in your hands to increase range of movement.

1 Place an elastic band around the tips of your fingers and thumb.

2 Slowly open your hand and move your fingers apart.

Variation: Use putty instead of elastic bands.

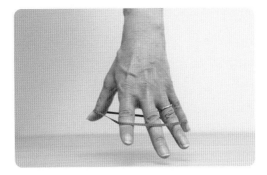

gentle movement in warm or cold water
During a flare-up, it is important to keep your hands and feet moving to maintain joint movement. Using bowls of cold water (or warm if you prefer) when your joints are hot and swollen will help with the pain and swelling as you exercise the joints gently.

wrist lifts

You can do this exercise with or without a weight. It is easy to progress or reduce, so you can keep your joints active when you are in pain. You can either use small dumbbells for this exercise or a bottle.

1 Sit with your elbows resting on a table.

2 Hold the weight in one hand. If using a bottle, grip the neck with the bottom of the bottle facing the ceiling.

3 Slowly move your hand so the palm is facing upwards and then downwards.

4 Only move the weight as far as you can control and without pain.

Repeat 10 times in each hand for one set, and do 2 sets.

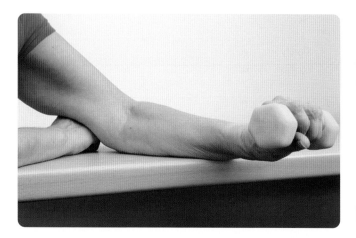

wrist lifts with resistance

Resistance bands and weights are also great for strengthening the wrists.

1 Support your elbow and forearm on a table and let your wrist drop over the edge.

2 Put a resistance band around the back of your hand or hold a weight.

3 Lift your wrist as high as you can while holding the weight in your hand or holding the band with the other hand.

Do 2 sets of 5–10 repetitions.

This exercise can be done with both sides of your forearm on the table to strengthen both sides of the wrist.

1   Place both your forearms with palms down on a table.

2   Hold a resistance band around both hands.

3   Slowly pull against the band and move your wrists sideways, keeping the palms face down on the table.

Do 2 sets of 5–10 repetitions.

trunk and low back

transverse abdominis

This is one of the most important exercises that you can learn if you have arthritis affecting your back. It may be a slow and dull exercise, but it is important to master it.

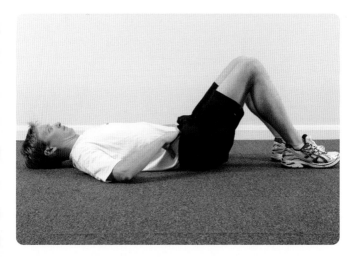

1 Lie on your back with your knees bent, your feet on the floor and your head supported on a small pillow or folded towel.

2 Relax the weight of your head and lengthen the back of your neck by reaching the top of your head towards the wall behind you.

3 Gently draw your shoulder blades down towards your waist to relax your neck and shoulders.

4 Place your feet and knees hip distance apart and gently place your finger tips on your lower tummy.

5 Imagine your pelvis is a bucket of water. Tip it backwards to spill some water out of the back of the bucket and you will feel your back gently flatten onto the mat.

6 Now tip it forwards to spill some water out of the front of the bucket and you will feel your lower back arch slightly.

7 Find your 'neutral spine' position by resting the bucket halfway between these two movements.

8 Maintaining this neutral spine position, take a breath in, then slowly breathe out until you have no breath left.

9 At the end of your out breath you will feel your deep abdominal muscles engage.

10 Gently maintain this muscle activation as you keep breathing in and out for up to ten breaths.

the cat stretch

This is a gentle exercise that you can do even when you have severe pain in your hips and back. It will help restore movement to your spine and release muscle spasm.

1 Kneel on all fours with your knees hip distance apart, and your hands shoulder width apart.

2 Imagine your pelvis is a bucket filled with water.

3 Tilt your pelvis forwards and backwards as if you are tipping water out of the front and the back of the bucket.

4 Ensure that you keep your spine straight and that all the movement comes from your pelvis and the bottom of your spine.

There is no limit on how many times you can do this exercise – it is gentle and can be repeated little and often.

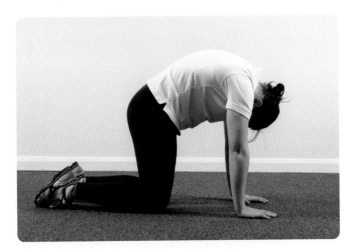

pole dancing

These are great for keeping the back and pelvis loose, and are a good place to start when you have a flare-up of your symptoms. You can do all the drills sitting, standing, kneeling on all fours and lying down, so they are versatile for all abilities and levels of pain. For standing position:

1 Stand with your hands on your hips and your feet hip distance apart, keeping your knees soft and slightly bent.

2 Imagine your pelvis is a bucket filled with water.

3 Ensure that you keep your spine straight and that all the movement comes from your pelvis and the bottom of your spine.

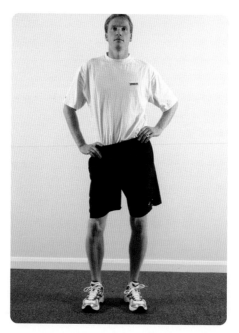

4 Then try any or all of the following:

● **Pelvic tilts:** tilt your pelvis forwards and backwards as if you are tipping water out of the front and the back of the bucket.
● **Side tilts:** tilt your pelvis side to side as if you are tipping water out of the left and right sides of the bucket.
● **Pelvic circles:** combining the pelvic and side tilts, put your hands on your hips and circle your pelvis as if you are swilling water around the top of the bucket but not letting any spill out.

Variations: Use whichever position is most comfortable for you, but aim to be able to do this exercise sitting or standing.

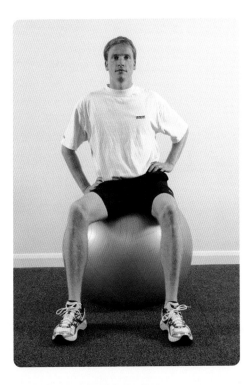

hips and knees

squats

If you have arthritis, your lifting technique is probably not as good as it could be, and squats are a great way to strengthen your legs to help you lift properly, making sure you don't hurt your knees. If your joints are sore or you are unfit, you can start by gently standing and carefully sitting back down in a chair. You can progress this exercise as you become stronger.

For instructions and photos see page 66. Repeat 5–10 times for one set, and do 3 sets. Rest as you need to between sets.

step-ups

Follow the instructions on page 64. Repeat each leg 10 times for each of 3 sets.

Variation: if your joints are sore and inflamed and you can't step up, march on the spot, lifting your foot to the height of the step or lower if you need to. You will soon be able to step up.

knee extension 1

This is an easy exercise to do to maintain range of movement in your knee joints when you are having a flare-up. You can even do it with an ice pack on your knee.

1 Sit on the floor with your back supported and your legs out in front of you.

2 Place a rolled towel under each knee.

3 Press the back of your left knee into the rolled towel and straighten the knee, lifting your heel off the floor.

4 Hold for 5 seconds.

5 Repeat with your right leg.

Do 3 sets of 10 repetitions.

Variation: You can make this harder by placing weights around your ankles. You can buy weights that fasten around the ankle with Velcro from most sports shops.

knee extension 2

This is also a great exercise to do during and after a flare-up.

1 Sit in a chair with your back supported.

2 Slowly lift your left foot off the floor and straighten your knee.

3 Hold for 5 seconds, then lower the foot back to the floor.

4 Repeat with your right leg.

Do 3 sets of 10 repetitions.

Variation: You can make this harder by using ankle weights (see above).

the clam

This is a great exercise to strengthen your buttocks and help control the movement and position of the hip.

1 Lie on your side with the arm underneath you comfortably placed by your head.

2 Rest your head on this arm if this is comfortable for your shoulder and elbow.

3 Bend your hips and knees up to about 90 degrees and rest your top hand on the floor.

4 Breathe out and lift your top knee upwards, keeping your feet together. You should feel this stretch in your buttock.

5 Breathe in and lower your top knee onto your bottom leg.

Repeat 10 times for one set. As you get stronger you can add extra sets.

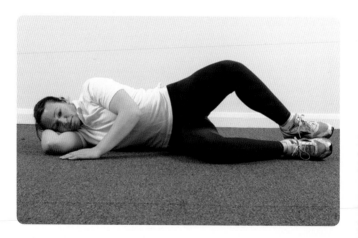

knees open and close

This is a gentle resistance band exercise which works the muscles that support your hip joints. It is easy to do even if you are having a flare-up.

1 Sit on a chair.

2 Put a resistance band around your knees.

3 Slowly open your knees as wide as your hips, and then slowly bring them back together.

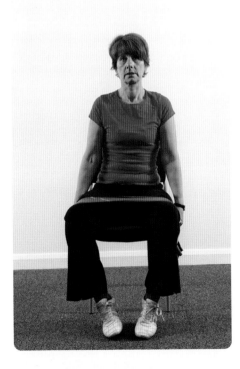

feet and ankles

foot intrinsics

This is a great exercise that you can do when watching TV or even sitting at your desk at work.

1 Take your shoes off and place your feet on a tissue or a towel.

2 Use your toes to claw at the tissue or towel, pulling it back until it is under the arch of your foot.

You can do a similar exercise when you are standing at the bus stop or in the supermarket queue by gripping the inside of your shoe.

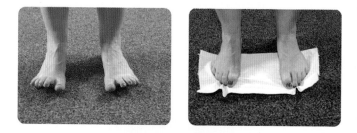

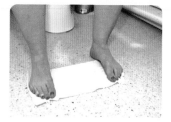

ankle circles

This is another exercise to do at any time when you are sitting down, or even in the bath or swimming pool, and can also be done during a flare-up.

1 Sit comfortably with your legs stretched out in front of you.

2 Point your toes, and imagine you are drawing circles, letters or your name in the air.

There is no limit on how many times you repeat this exercise – little and often is a good goal.

Variation: To make this more difficult, loop a resistance band around your foot and hold the ends in your hand.

heel raises

This is a great exercise to strengthen your calf muscles and make you stronger for increasing your daily walking sessions. If the small joints of your feet are painful, make sure you are wearing comfortable shoes and/or standing on a soft rug or carpet.

1 Start in standing position – if you need help to balance, hold on to the back of a chair or the kitchen worktop.

2 Slowly lift your heels off the floor, and then lower them back down again.

Do 2 sets of 5–10 repetitions.

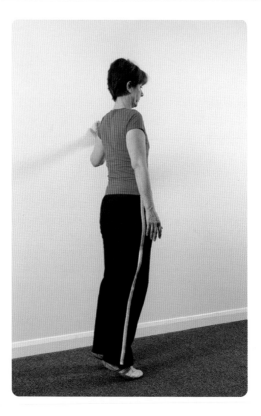

balance exercises

These are great exercises to strengthen your ankles and improve your balance. It is specifically important to do them if you have chronic swelling and weakness caused by your arthritis or due to a flare-up. Swelling around the ankle joint will make the muscles weak and more prone to sprains.

balancing on a wobble cushion

You can buy wobble cushions from exercise equipment shops or online from www.physiosupplies.co.uk. For this exercise you can even use an inflatable mattress to create an unstable surface to balance on.

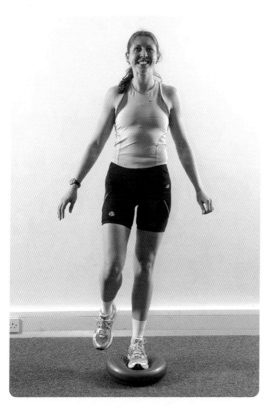

1 Stand with both feet on the wobble cushion, keeping your knees soft. Allow yourself to wobble a little, as the point of the exercise is to control the wobble without falling off the cushion.

2 You may need to place the cushion near a wall or kitchen worktop to help you balance – when you get stronger you will be able to balance without support.

3 To make it harder, stand on one leg.

4 You can practise standing on one leg every time you clean your teeth – a great way to make it a daily exercise with very little effort.

ankle flicks

This exercise will help with ankle strength, but will also really help your balance and help prevent falls. All you need is a tennis ball and a wall.

1 Stand on one leg next to a wall.

2 Using a tennis ball, kick the ball with the side of your foot against the wall.

3 You can work the muscles on the inside and the outside of your ankle by a simple change of position and kicking with the inner or outer part of the foot.

4 You can do a similar exercise using a resistance band, so you can still do the exercise if your arthritis means you need to sit down.

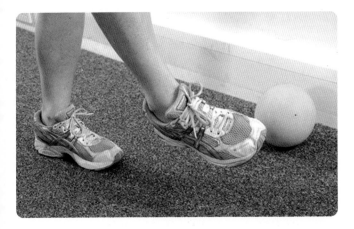

As you become stronger at the ankle and get used to exercising the joint, it will start to feel less stiff and more comfortable as a result.

find out more

osteoarthritis
Arthritis Care
www.arthritiscare.org.uk

Arthritis Research Campaign
www.arc.org.uk

rheumatoid arthritis
National Rheumatoid Arthritis Society
www.rheumatoid.org.uk
Freephone helpline 9.30-4.30 Monday-Friday 0800 298 7650

exercise equipment and assistance aids
Aids to Mobility (links to other websites)
www.aidstomobility.org

Help My Mobility (product buying tips)
www.help-my-mobility.co.uk

Physio Supplies
www.physiosupplies.co.uk

Drug treatments
www.besthealth.bmj.com

pain management
The Pain Society
www.britishpainsociety.org.uk

CBT
British Association for Cognitive and Behavioural Therapists
http://www.babcp.com

Mood Gym
http://moodgym.anu.edu.au

Living Life to the Full
www.livinglifetothefull.com

return to work
The Equality and Human Rights Commission
www.equalityhumanrights.com

Expert Patients Programmes
www.expertpatients.co.uk

acupuncture and yoga
Acupuncture Association of Chartered Physiotherapists
www.aacp.org.uk

British Medical Acupuncture Society
www.medical-acupuncture.co.uk

Triyoga
www.triyoga.co.uk

complimentary therapies
You can download a useful booklet from ARC
www.arc.org.uk